Pushpa Raj Joshi

Mitochondrial DNA abnormalities in patients with idiopathic myositis

Pushpa Raj Joshi

Mitochondrial DNA abnormalities in patients with idiopathic myositis

Molecular, histological and biochemical analysis

Südwestdeutscher Verlag für Hochschulschriften

Impressum / Imprint
Bibliografische Information der Deutschen Nationalbibliothek: Die Deutsche Nationalbibliothek verzeichnet diese Publikation in der Deutschen Nationalbibliografie; detaillierte bibliografische Daten sind im Internet über http://dnb.d-nb.de abrufbar.
Alle in diesem Buch genannten Marken und Produktnamen unterliegen warenzeichen-, marken- oder patentrechtlichem Schutz bzw. sind Warenzeichen oder eingetragene Warenzeichen der jeweiligen Inhaber. Die Wiedergabe von Marken, Produktnamen, Gebrauchsnamen, Handelsnamen, Warenbezeichnungen u.s.w. in diesem Werk berechtigt auch ohne besondere Kennzeichnung nicht zu der Annahme, dass solche Namen im Sinne der Warenzeichen- und Markenschutzgesetzgebung als frei zu betrachten wären und daher von jedermann benutzt werden dürften.

Bibliographic information published by the Deutsche Nationalbibliothek: The Deutsche Nationalbibliothek lists this publication in the Deutsche Nationalbibliografie; detailed bibliographic data are available in the Internet at http://dnb.d-nb.de.
Any brand names and product names mentioned in this book are subject to trademark, brand or patent protection and are trademarks or registered trademarks of their respective holders. The use of brand names, product names, common names, trade names, product descriptions etc. even without a particular marking in this works is in no way to be construed to mean that such names may be regarded as unrestricted in respect of trademark and brand protection legislation and could thus be used by anyone.

Coverbild / Cover image: www.ingimage.com

Verlag / Publisher:
Südwestdeutscher Verlag für Hochschulschriften
ist ein Imprint der / is a trademark of
AV Akademikerverlag GmbH & Co. KG
Heinrich-Böcking-Str. 6-8, 66121 Saarbrücken, Deutschland / Germany
Email: info@svh-verlag.de

Herstellung: siehe letzte Seite /
Printed at: see last page
ISBN: 978-3-8381-3376-8

Zugl. / Approved by: Halle, MLU, Diss., 2011

Copyright © 2012 AV Akademikerverlag GmbH & Co. KG
Alle Rechte vorbehalten. / All rights reserved. Saarbrücken 2012

Dedicated to my Dad, Mamu and my beloved wife Reshma

Table of contents

1.	**Introduction**	**1**
1.1	Mitochondria	1
1.2	Mitochondrial genetics	3
1.3	Mitochondrial DNA mutations	5
1.4	Common features of mtDNA deletions	9
1.5	Generation of mtDNA deletions	14
1.6	Histological changes in mitochondrial disease	19
1.7	Forms of myositis	20
1.7.1	Dermatomyositis	21
1.7.2	Polymyositis	24
1.7.3	Inclusion body myositis	26
2.	**Background of the study**	**31**
2.1	Inclusion body myositis and mtDNA deletions	32
2.2	Polymyositis/dermatomyositis and mtDNA deletions	33
3.	**Patients**	**35**
3.1	Myositis patients	35
3.2	Normal controls	37
4.	**Materials and Methods**	**38**
4.1	Materials	38
4.2	Methods	39
4.2.1	Extraction of DNA from muscle	39
4.2.2	Qualitative analysis: mtDNA deletions	41

4.2.2.1	Long range PCR	41
4.2.2.1.1	Modification of long range PCR	41
4.2.2.2	Common deletion PCR	44
4.2.2.3	Southern-blot analysis	46
4.2.3	Quantitative analysis: mtDNA common deletion	47
4.2.3.1	Real-time PCR analysis	47
4.2.3.1.1	Implementation of real-time PCR in present study	49
4.2.4	Control of real time PCR protocol	51
4.2.5	Multiple-cell real-time PCR	51
4.2.5.1	COX/SDH staining	52
4.2.5.2	Dissection of single cells and DNA extraction	52
4.2.6	Biochemical enzyme activity	53
4.2.6.1	Citrate synthase activity	53
4.2.6.2	COX activity	54
5.	**Results**	**56**
5.1	Molecular genetic findings	56
5.1.1	Long-Range-PCR	56
5.1.2	Common deletion PCR	56
5.1.3	Real-time PCR common deletion	57
5.1.4	Multiple-cell real-time PCR: common deletion	60
5.1.5	Level of common deletion in CPEO patients	60
5.2	Biochemical results	61
5.3	Comparison of different mitochondrial abnormalities	62
6.	**Statistical Analysis**	**63**

6.1	Comparison of levels of common deletion in CPEO patients in Southern-blot and real-time PCR	63
6.2	2x2 Contingency tables comparing mtDNA abnormalities	63
6.3	Comparison of degree of heteroplasmy of the common deletion	65
6.4	Scatter plots	65
6.5	Correlation analysis	70
6.6	Statistical comparison of molecular and histological changes	70
7.	**Discussion**	71
8.	**Conclusions**	84
9.	**References**	85
	Appendix	105
	Theses	113
	Acknowledgement	116

List of abbrevations

ALT:	Alanine transaminase
ANOVA:	Analysis of variance
ATP:	Adenosine tri-phosphate
bp:	Base pairs
BSA:	Bovine serum albumin
CD:	Common deletion
CK:	Creatine kinase
CNF:	Cytochrome c oxidase negative fibres
CoA	Coenzyme A
COX:	Cytochrome c oxidase
CPEO:	Chronic progressive external opthalmoplegia
CS:	Citrate synthase
DAB:	Diaminobenzidine
DIG:	Digoxigenin
DM:	Dermatomyositis
DNA:	Deoxyribonucleic acid
dNTP:	deoxy- Nucleotide triphosphates
DSB:	Double strand break
DTNB	2-nitobenzoic acid
DTT:	Dimethiothreitol
ECL kit:	Enhanced chemoluminescence analysis kit
EM:	Electron microscopy
EMG:	Electromyograph
F:	Female

FAD:	Flavine adenine dinucleotide (Oxidised)
$FADH_2$:	Flavine adenine dinucleotide (Reduced)
FRET:	Fluorescence resonance energy transfer
HE:	Hematoxylin and eosin
HIV:	Human immunodeficiency virus
HTLV-1:	Human T-lymphocyte virus-1
HVR2:	Human variable region 2
IBM:	Inclusion body myositis
kb:	Kilo base
KCl:	Potassium chloride
KSS:	Kearns-Sayre syndrome
LDH:	Lactate dehydrogenase
LHON:	Leber's hereditary optic neuropathy
M:	Male
MELAS:	Mitochondrial encephalomyopathy lactic acidosis and stroke like episodes
MERRF:	Myoclonic epilepsy with ragged-red fibres
MRC:	Medical research council
mt:	Mitochondrial
mtDNA:	Mitochondrial deoxyribonucleic acid
MUAP:	Motor unit action potential
MW:	Molecular weight
$Na_2H_2PO_4$:	Sodium bi-phosphate
NAD^+:	Nicotinamide adenine dinucleotide (Oxidised)
NADH:	Nicotinamide adenine dinucleotide (Reduced)
NBT:	Nitro blue tetrazolium

ND1:	NADH dehydrogenase subunit 1
ND4:	NADH dehydrogenase subunit 4
ND5:	NADH dehydrogenase subunit 5
O_H:	Origin of replication of the heavy strand
O_L:	Origin of replication of the light strand
OriZ:	Zone of replication
OXPHOS:	Oxidative phosphorylation
PCR:	Polymerase chain reaction
PM:	Polymyositis
PMS:	Phenazine methosulphate
POLG:	Polymerase gamma
PS:	Pearson syndrome
RITOLS:	Ribonucleotide incorporation throughout the lagging strand
rpm:	Rotations per minute
RNA:	Ribonucleic acid
RRF:	Ragged-red fibres
rRNA:	Ribosomal ribonucleic acid
SDH:	Succinate dehydrogenase
SGPT:	Serum glutamic pyruvic transaminase
Sig.:	Significance
SYBR:	Synergy Brands Inc.
Taq:	*Thermus aquiticus*
TF:	Tubular filaments
TIM:	Translocase of the inner membrane
TOM:	Translocase of the outer membrane

Tris-HCL:	Tris Hydrochloric acid
tRNA:	Transfer ribonucleic acid
U:	Units
V:	Volts

1. Introduction

1.1 Mitochondria

Mitochondria occupy a substantial portion of the cytoplasmic volume of eucaryotic cells and they have been essential for the evolution of complex animals. During conversion of pyruvate from glucose via glycolysis, only a small fraction of total free energy is released. The complete metabolism of sugars takes place within the mitochondria where the end product of glycolysis, the pyruvate, is imported and is oxidized to carbon dioxide and water. Mitochondria are usually known to be stiff, elongated cylindrical structures with a diameter of 0.5-1 micrometer, resembling bacteria. Time-lapse microcinematography of living cells, however, shows that mitochondria are remarkably mobile and plastic organelles, constantly changing their shape and even fusing with one another and then separating again [Suelmann and Fischer, 2000].

Each mitochondrion contains a unique collection of proteins. Most of these 1000 or so different mitochondrial proteins are encoded in the nucleus and imported into the mitochondrion from the cytoplasm by specialized protein translocases of the outer (TOM, translocase of the outer membrane) and inner (TIM) mitochondrial membrane.

The outer mitochondrial membrane contains many porin molecules, a type of transport protein that forms large aqueous channels through the lipid bi-layer, which is permeable to all molecules of 5000 daltons or less, including small proteins. Such molecules can enter the intermembrane space, but most of them cannot pass the impermeable inner membrane. Thus, whereas the intermembrane space is chemically equivalent to cytosol with respect to the small molecules it contains, the matrix contains a highly selected set of these molecules.

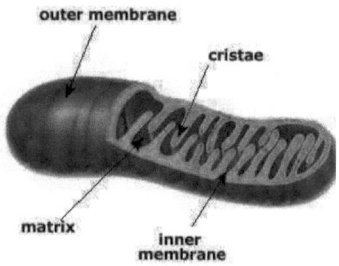

Figure 1: Mitochondria with inner and outer membranes (http://click4biology.info)

The major working part of the mitochondrion, the inner membrane is highly specialized. The lipid bi-layer contains a high proportion of the 'double' phospholipids cardiolipin, which has four fatty acids rather than two and may help to make the membrane especially impermeable to ions. This membrane also contains a variety of transport proteins that make it selectively permeable to those small molecules that are metabolized or required by the many mitochondrial enzymes concentrated in the matrix. The matrix enzymes include those that metabolize pyruvate and fatty acids to produce acetyl CoA and those that oxidize acetyl CoA in the citric acid cycle. The principle end products of this oxidation are CO_2, which is released from the cell as waste, and NADH, which is the main source of electrons for transport along the respiratory chain – the name given to the electron-transport chain in mitochondria. The enzymes of the respiratory chain are embedded in the inner mitochondrial membrane, they are essential to the process of oxidative phosphorylation, which generates most of the animal cell's ATP.

Mitochondria can use both pyruvate and fatty acids as fuel. Pyruvate comes from glucose and other sugars, whereas fatty acids come from fats. Both of these fuel molecules are transported across the inner membrane and then are converted to the crucial metabolic intermediate acetyl CoA by enzymes located in the mitochondrial matrix. The acetyl groups in acetyl CoA are then oxidized in the mitochondrial matrix via the citric acid cycle. The cycle converts the carbon atoms in acetyl CoA to CO_2, which the cell releases as a waste product. Most importantly, the oxidation generates high-energy electrons, carried by the activated carrier molecules NADH and $FADH_2$. These high-energy molecules are then transferred to the inner mitochondrial membrane, where they enter the electron-transport chain; the loss of electrons from NADH and $FADH_2$ also regenerates the NAD^+ and FAD that is needed for continued oxidative metabolism.

1.2 Mitochondrial genetics:

Mitochondria are the only sub-cellular organelles that contain their own genetic material. Until 1963, there was no knowledge about the mitochondrial DNA (mtDNA). MtDNA is exclusively maternally inherited, has its own genetic code, and has virtually no introns. The nucleotide sequence was fully described in 1981 and is found to encode

13 structural components of the respiratory chain/OXPHOS system, 22 transfer RNAs (tRNAs), and 2 ribosomal RNAs (rRNAs) [Anderson et al., 1981]. The presence of multiple copies of the mitochondrial genome leads to the phenomenon of heteroplasmy, in which differing proportions of mutant and wild-type mtDNA coexist in the mitochondria of a cell. This means that mitochondrial genetics bears greater similarities to population genetics than to traditional Mendelian genetics.

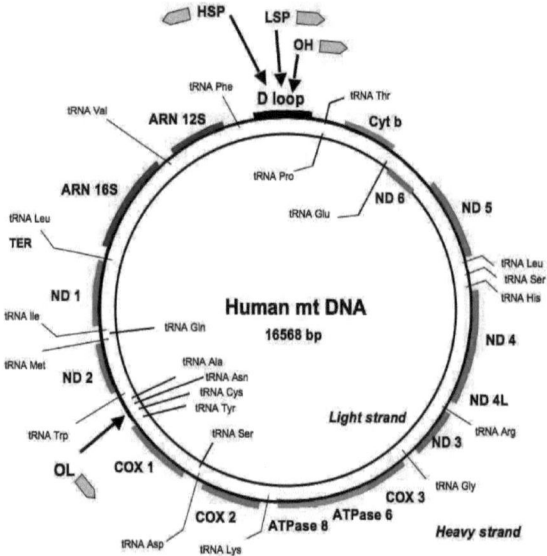

Figure 2: The human mitochondrial DNA (mtDNA) [Nadege et al., 2009]

The study of mtDNA is quite fascinating due to its unique genetic role in human diseases. The first pathogenic mutations of mtDNA were identified in 1988 in patients with Leber hererditary optic neuropathy (LHON) and chronic progressive external ophthalmoplegia (CPEO) [Holt et al., 1988; Wallace et al., 1988]. Since then it has become increasingly clear that the defects of this diminutive genome are an important cause of neurological diseases. The most common mitochondrial genetic defects that are seen in individuals with mtDNA-associated diseases are point mutations and large-scale deletions.

1.3 Mitochondrial DNA mutations

Mutations in mtDNA can be distinguished between point mutations and large-scale rearrangements. Point mutations are frequently inherited maternally and are associated with mitochondrial syndromes such as mitochondrial encephalomyopathy lactic acidosis and stroke like episodes (MELAS), Myoclonic epilepsy with ragged-red fibres (MERRF) or Leber hererditary optic neuropathy (LHON). Point mutations are frequently present in heteroplasmy. However, homoplasmic pathogenic point mutations were increasingly described during the last years [McFarland et al., 2007]. More than 200 pathogenic mtDNA point mutations have been described [Servidei, 2003], in addition to a large number of deletion species. Much is still unknown regarding the molecular pathogenesis of these mutations. However, despite many detailed studies, it is still difficult to explain the lack of correlation between genotype and phenotype for many mtDNA mutations. Some variations in phenotype have been, however, explained due to differing tissue distributions of heteroplasmic mutations or polymorphisms [Lertrit et al., 1994; Holt et al., 1997], immunological mechanisms [Harding et al., 1992], and environmental factors [Prezant et al., 1993].

Large-scale rearrangements of the mitochondrial genome are always heteroplasmic and may involve single or multiple deletions or partial duplications. The clinical phenotypes most commonly associated with these mutations are chronic progressive external opthalmoplegia (CPEO), the Kearns-Sayre (KSS) and Pearson syndromes (PS) [Moraes et al., 1989; Holt et al., 1989 (a)]. There is no obvious relationship between the clinical phenotype, size, location, or percentage of the mtDNA deletion(s) in muscle. However, the proportion of deleted mtDNA molecules varies widely between tissues, and tissue distribution and segregation is likely to be important in determining the phenotype. Studies report that the mitochondrial disorders are induced when the concentration of mtDNA deletions is 30% and greater in muscle tissue [Holt et al., 1988; Moraes et al., 1989]. Evolution of a phenotype may be explained by selection against deleted mtDNA molecules in rapidly dividing tissues, such as bone marrow, paralleled by accumulation of deleted molecules in non-dividing tissues, such as muscle and the central nervous system [Larson et al., 1990].

Although many different mtDNA deletion molecules have been described, ranging in size from 1 to 10 kb, 30-40% of all these deletions are identical, spanning 4977 bp from ATPase 8 to ND5 and flanked by a perfect 13-bp direct repeat [Holt et al., 1989 (b)]. Single deletions are usually sporadic, although they may occasionally be maternally inherited

[Bernes et al., 1993; Chinnery et al., 2004]. They are present at low levels in human oocytes [Chen et al., 1995], but transmission is thought to be prevented in many cases by the bottleneck effect [Brown, 1997]. Multiple deletions are, however, inherited as Mendelian traits, either recessive or dominant. The first reported example of Mendelian trait associated with lesions of human mitochondrial genome, genetic analysis indicated that in a large Italian family, containing several individuals affected by late-onset mitochondrial myopathy, both the clinical picture and the mtDNA deletions are produced by an autosomal dominant mechanism [Zeviani et al., 1989]. The study rules out the maternal inheritance by the recurrent transmission of the clinical and the molecular traits to patrilinear descendants. Additionally, no same breakpoints in PCR-clones of different individuals were found suggesting that the heteroplasmic mtDNA populations are not transmitted *per se*, but are rather generated *de novo* by a common mechanism [Zeviani et al., 1989].

The mechanism of pathogenesis of deletions is thought to be via impaired mitochondrial translation, and this has been supported by cybrid studies. Impaired mitochondrial translation has been observed in transmitochondrial cybrids containing 60% or more deleted mtDNA [Hayashi et al., 1991]. Single-fibre analysis of muscle from patients with mtDNA deletions, demonstrating a higher percentage of deleted mtDNA in COX-negative fibres compared with COX-positive fibres, also provides evidence from impaired mitochondrial translation secondary to the deletion [Mita et al., 1989]. Impairment of mitochondrial translation most probably follows insufficiency of tRNAs that is due to deletion of tRNA genes.

Duplications are seen in KSS and PS and in patients with diabetes and deafness [Poulton et al., 1989; Supreti-Furga et al., 1993; Dunbar et al., 1993]. Maternal inheritance of duplications has been reported [Ballinger et al., 1992; Rötig et al., 1992; Supreti-Furga et al., 1993; Dunbar et al., 1993]. The pathogenic mechanism of duplications is uncertain, but those involving the D-loop may interfere with the binding and function of *trans*-acting nuclear factors. However, there is much controversy regarding whether duplications are intrinsically pathogenic [Manfredi et al., 1997].

MtDNA deletions are known to have an important role in human pathology in three different clinical scenarios: first, single mtDNA deletions are a common cause of sporadic mitochondrial diseases; in these cases, an identical mtDNA deletion is detected in all cells within an affected tissue [Schaefer et al., 2008]. Second, in another large group of individuals with mitochondrial diseases, multiple mtDNA deletions are identified in affected tissue, particularly in the muscle and the central nervous system [Taylor and Turnbull, 2005]. Third, deletions of mtDNA have been identified in aged postmitotic tissues and individuals with other disease such as neurodegenerative diseases and toxic myopathie due to ziduvudine [Dalakas et al., 1990]. However, the level of mtDNA deletions is often much lower than that seen in individuals with mitochondrial diseases [Bender et al., 2006; Kraytsberg et al., 2006].

1.4 Common features of mtDNA deletions

Most mtDNA deletions share similar characteristics: most are located in the major arc between two proposed origins of replication (O_H and O_L; mitomap) and are predominantly flanked by short direct repeats [Samuels et al., 2004; Bua et al., 2006]. Studies show, there are two distinct regions in mtDNA that are related directly with mtDNA deletions: the ND1 region, where the DNA is found to be rarely deleted and the ND4 region, where the DNA is found to be frequently deleted. A study reports that in ND1 region deletions were seen in only 6% in cases with single deletion and no deletion in cases with multiple deletions. Contrastingly, in the ND4 region, deletions were reported in 82% of the cases with large scale deletion and 96% cases with multiple deletions [He et al., 2002]. A recent study reports that the mtDNA-deletion characteristics are similar under all circumstances with no notable difference in size, presence or absence of flanking repeat sequences or lengths of repeats suggesting that a similar mechanism should be generating the mtDNA deletions in different clinical situations [Krishnan et al., 2008].

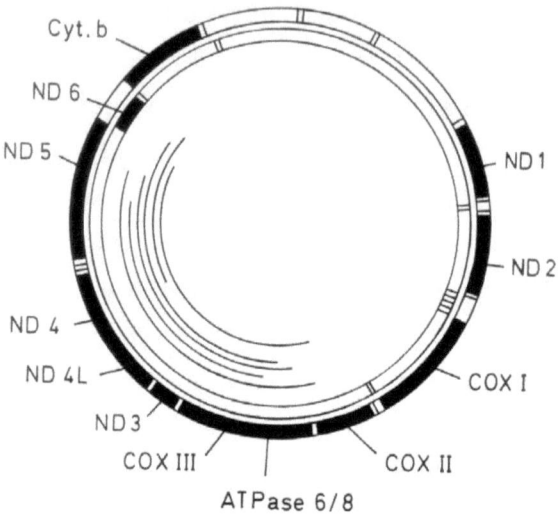

Figure 3: Mitochondrial deletions in patients with CPEO. All the deletions are featured in the ND4 region [Gerbitz, Zierz, et al., 1990]

It has been considered that replication is the likely mechanism behind deletion formation. Two main models for mtDNA replication are proposed: a strand-asynchronous (strand-displacement) mode of replication [Robberson et al., 1972; Yasukawa et al., 2006], and a more conventional coupled leading-lagging-strand replication [Holt et al., 2000]. The observation that most reported mtDNA deletions occur in the major arc has led to the proposal that mtDNA deletions could be generated through a slipped-strand replication mechanism [Schoffner et al., 1989]. This mechanism, however, largely assumes the asynchronous mode of replication, as it predicts large regions of single-stranded DNA. On the other hand, recent modifications of the strand-displacement model argue that large regions of single-stranded DNA do not exist, rather, the lagging-strand template is largely protected by RNA [Yang et al., 2002; Yasukawa et al., 2006].

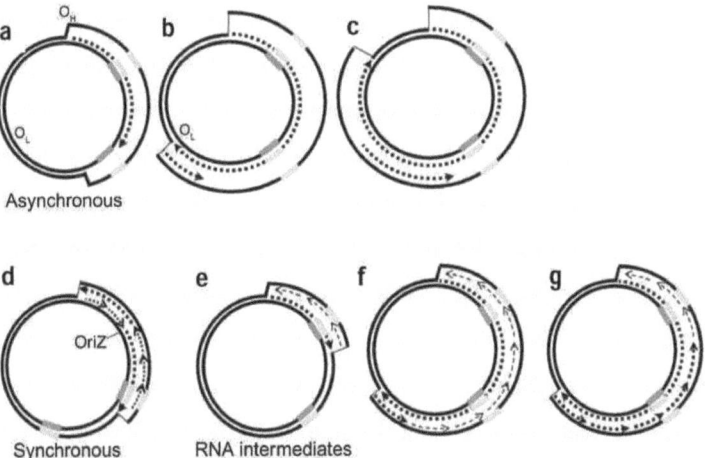

Figure 4: (a–c) Asynchronous method of replication of mtDNA (a) Replication begins in the D loop at the O_H, displacing the light strand from the heavy strand. (b,c) Replication of the light strand begins in the opposite direction until both strands have been fully replicated. (d) Replication begins from a zone of replication (OriZ) on the genome and replicates initially bidirectionally via conventional coupled leading- and lagging-strand synthesis. (e–g) Alternatively, the ribonucleotide incorporation throughout the lagging strand (RITOLS) model of replication initiates in the noncoding region close to O_H, displacing the light strand from the heavy strand. [Krishnan et al., 2008].

Although replication remains a favored model for explaining the generation of mtDNA deletions, there are some concerns. For example, for mtDNA deletions to occur as proposed, mtDNA would need to be not only actively replicating, but replicating at the point where the single-stranded 5' and 3' repeats come together to form a loop when the strand break occurs. In postmitotic cells, the rate of mitochondrial turnover is unknown, but it is thought to be low, possibly in the order of days [Wang et al., 1997]. If replication is the principle mechanism underlying the generation of mtDNA deletions, then in mitotic cells where mtDNA replication is more frequent, there should be a greater chance of mtDNA deletions occurring. Although mtDNA deletions might be rapidly selected against in dividing cells, a study shows that in human colonic tissue, there is very little evidence of selection, yet no deleted mtDNA molecules were detected, despite an exhaustive search [Taylor et al., 2003]. Another factor crucial for the viability of the slipped-strand replication model is the retention of the 3'-repeat sequence, as the model predicts that strand slippage can only occur during replication of the nascent H strand with dissociation of the lagging L strand. However, it has been found that mtDNA deletions in neuronal and muscle cells where the 3' repeat is lost (47% and 75% of all imperfect repeat breakpoints analyzed, respectively) [Bua et al., 2006; Reeve et al., 2008].

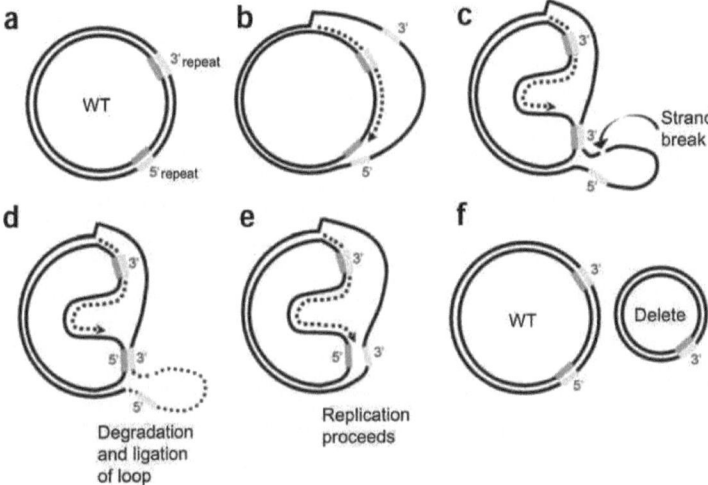

Figure 5*: mtDNA deletion through a slipped-strand model of replication (a) An mtDNA molecule indicating the presence of two direct repeats labeled 5' and 3'. (b) Replication begins in the D loop from O_H, displacing the light strand from the heavy strand. (c) The single-stranded 3' repeat of the light strand mis-anneals with the newly exposed single-stranded 5' heavy-strand repeat, generating a downstream loop of the light strand. The single-stranded loop is susceptible to strand breaks. (d) The damaged loop is degraded until it reaches the double-strand regions, and ligation of the free ends of the heavy strand takes place. (e,f) Replication is resumed (e), leading to the production of a wild type and a deleted mtDNA molecule (f) [Krishnan et al., 2008].*

A strong reason for favoring replication as a mechanism of deletion formation has been the apparently high frequency of mtDNA deletions in the major arc of the mitochondrial genome. For mtDNA deletions to accumulate within a cell, it is essential that replication of the delete species occurs. As direct repeats are associated with most mtDNA deletions, a recent study reports to have identified all repeats 5–9 bp and ≥10 bp in length that occur throughout the human mtDNA genome and the possible number of mtDNA deletions that could be formed in the major or minor arcs or that spanned either or both the O_H or O_L were counted [Krishnan et al., 2008]. Excluding those repeat pairs that remove either the O_H or O_L, assuming these deleted molecules would be unable to replicate. The study hence suggest that the high frequency of mtDNA deletions in the major arc merely reflects the relative number of possible deletion-forming sites in the two arcs and does not indicate or support a particular mechanism underlying the generation of the deletions.

1.5 Generation of mtDNA deletions

The study proposes that mtDNA deletions are initiated by single-stranded regions of mtDNA generated through exonuclease activity at double-strand breaks [Krishnan et al., 2008]. These single strands would then be free to anneal with microhomologous sequences [Haber, 2000], such as repeat sequences (including homopolymeric runs) on other single-stranded mtDNA or within the noncoding region. Once annealed, subsequent repair, ligation and degradation of the remaining exposed single strands would result in the formation of an intact mitochondrial genome harboring a deleted portion. The 16070-bp region in human mtDNA is known to be a hotspot for deletion formation, most likely because of its single-stranded nature within the D loop. This observation could provide additional support for the importance of single-stranded regions in the formation of mtDNA deletions. Another explanation for the deletion hotspot in this region comes from the previous suggestion that the 16070 region may form a boundary at which replication fork arrest occurs [Bowmaker et al., 2003; Wanrooji et al., 2004]. This scenario itself explains why a large number of mtDNA deletions have breakpoints in this region, as it is possible that exonuclease activity acting on the DSBs may be unable to degrade past this boundary point.

The mitochondrial DNA polymerase, POLG, has a well characterized 3→5 exonuclease activity [Hudson and Chinnery, 2006]; another potential candidate is SFN, the human homolog of *Escherichia coli* Orn and yeast Rex2(Ynt20). SFN shows 3→5 exonuclease activity for single-stranded RNA or DNA oligomers [Nguyen et al., 2000]. Ytn20 has been shown to be mitochondrially targeted [Blakely et al., 2004], and its human homolog, SFN, also has a putative N-terminal mitochondrial presequence and consensus cleavage site, consistent with a mitochondrial localization [Nguyen et al., 2000]. Although both of these potential candidates are capable of exoDNase activity, neither is likely to degrade large regions, such as those spanning the repeat sequences. However, evidence for dual targeting of mitochondrial proteins is becoming increasingly common, raising the possibility of mitochondrial localization for other 3→5 exoDNases, such as TREX1 or TREX2.

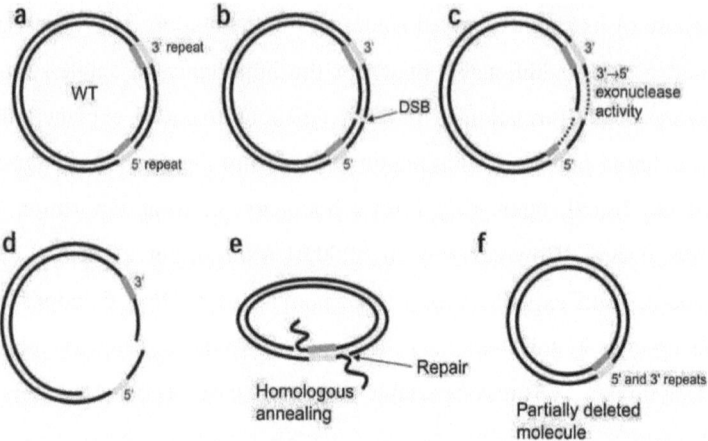

Figure 6: *Generation of mtDNA deletions during repair of DSBs. (a) An mtDNA molecule indicating the presence of two direct repeats, labeled 3' and 5'. (b) Production of a double-strand break. (c,d) The DSB is susceptible to 3'→5' exonuclease activity, leading to the production of single strands (d). (e) The 5'- and 3'-repeat sequences can misanneal, leading to degradation of the unbound single strands and ligation of the double strands. (f) This results in the production of a deleted mtDNA, which has copies of both the 5' and 3' repeats. If there are mismatched bases within the repeats, subsequent repair could use either strand as a template to correct the mismatch [Krishnan et al., 2008].*

Single, large-scale mtDNA deletions are a common cause of mitochondrial disease [Taylor and Turnbull, 2005]. In most cases, these mutations are sporadic [Chinnery et al., 2004], and previous studies have shown that these mutations are present in the oocyte [Blakely et al., 2004]. MtDNA is maintained in the mature oocyte for many years—indeed, until fertilization. As there is little—if any—mtDNA replication during this time, it seems unlikely that deletion formation occurs as a result of abnormalities in replication. It has been opined that it is very much likely that these deletions arise as a consequence of the repair of damaged mtDNA, through the same mechanism as that seen in other postmitotic cells, such as neurons and muscle [Krishnan et al., 2008].

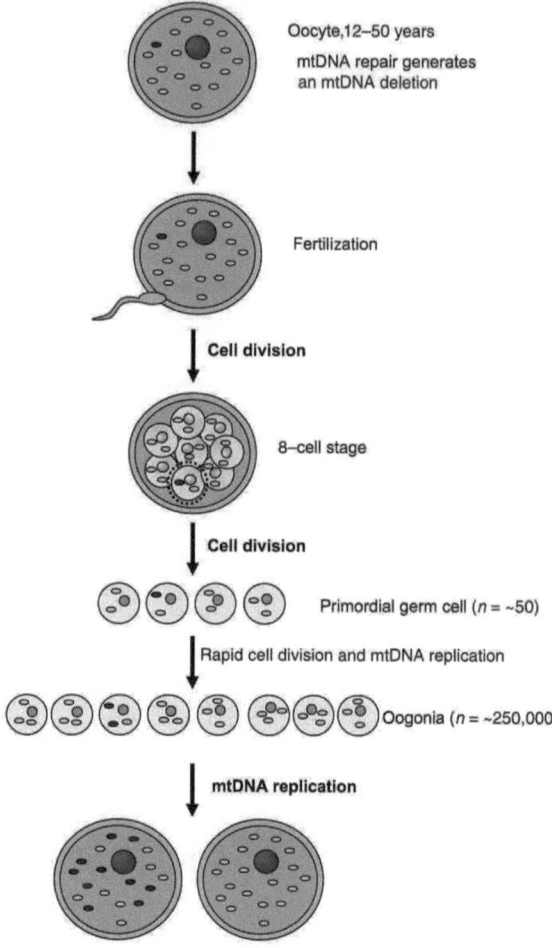

Figure 7: *Proposed model showing how sporadic mtDNA deletions occur in the oocyte. [Krishnan et al., 2008].*

There have been a number of studies providing evidence that low levels (<0.1%) of mtDNA deletions exist in human oocytes [Chen et al., 1995; Barritt et al., 1999; Chan et al., 2005]. If an oocyte containing an mtDNA deletion is fertilized, in most cases, the deletion will be selected against during embryo development through a bottleneck or other selection processes. However, in a small number of cases, the mtDNA deletion may be segregated to form primordial germ cells and escape the selection at the bottleneck, and it could go on to replicate and populate the oocyte. The female child born would thus be unaffected, and it would be the grandchild who would be at risk of being born with high levels of the pathogenic mtDNA deletion.

1.6 Histological changes in mitochondrial disease

Ragged-red fibres are the important histological markers of mitochondrial diseases and are present in large numbers in skeletal muscles of patients with mitochondrial myopathy and encephalomyopathy [DiMauro et al., 1993]. The ragged-red fibres are easily detected by Gomori trichome staining and often have absent or deficient COX activity [Hammans et al., 1992 (a)]. The fibres with absent or deficient COX activity are stained blue with modified COX/SDH staining in contrast to brown coloration of the normal fibres.

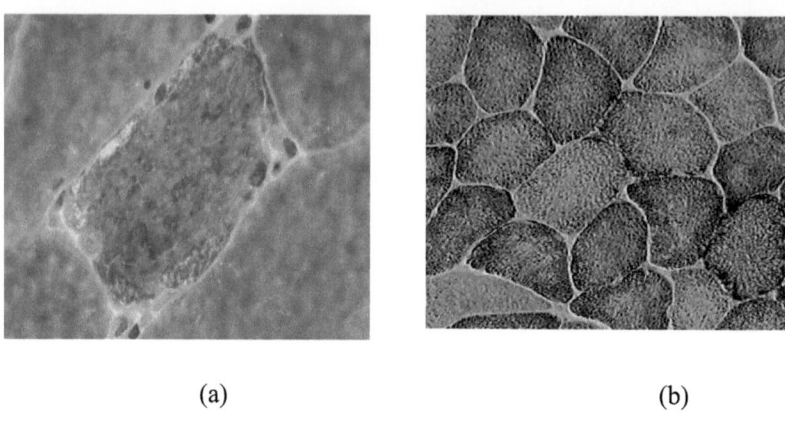

(a) (b)

Figures 8: (a) Gomori trichrome frozen section showing the classic ragged red fibre in the centre of the field. The peripheral rim of red staining represents aggregates of mitochondria and (b) cytochrome oxidase (COX) and succinic dehydrogenase (SDH) frozen section showing brown fibres stained with both COX and SDH activities and blue fibers that are stained only for SDH activity because of absence of COX activity. Several blue fibers have subsarcolemmal dense blue stain.

1.7 Forms of myositis

Myositis is an inflammatory autoimmune disease characterised by inflammation and weakness mainly of the proximal muscles. Dermatomyositis (DM), polymyositis (PM), and the inclusion body myositis (IBM) are three types of myositis depending on the location of the association of inflammation and weakness. In addition, some patients with myositis also have another autoimmune disease called as 'overlap syndrome'. The diseases most commonly associated are rheumatoid arthritis, lupus, scleroderma and Sjogren's syndrome. However, all forms of myositis involve chronic or persistent muscle inflammation. The muscle inflammation always results in weakness and less often in heat, swelling and pain of the muscles. Not only muscle but the myositis may be associated with inflammation in other organs like heart, lungs, intestine, skin and liver.

The inflammatory myopathies are auto-immune diseases, which means, the immune system of the body goes awry and attacks its own tissues. The environmental factors are believed to trigger these diseases in genetically susceptible individuals. The specific causes or triggering events of the inflammatory myopathies are unknown but viruses have been implicated.

These inflammatory myositis are clinically, histologically, and pathogenically distinct [Table 1] [Dalakas, 1991; Engel et al., 1994; Amato and Barohn, 1997]. The incidence of these disorders is very low, as low as 1 in 100000 [Medsger et al., 1970; Dalakas, 1991]. Although there are a few reports of DM, PM, and IBM occurring in parents and children and in siblings, including identical twins [Cook et al., 1963; Banker, 1975; Amato and Shebert, 1998], the inflammatory myopathies are best considered as acquired diseases.

1.7.1 Dermatomyositis

DM can present at any age but is common in childhood [Medsger et al., 1970; Bruguier et al., 1984]. Women are affected more commonly than men in both the childhood and adult onset forms. Onset of weakness is typically sub-acute (over several weeks), although it can develop abruptly (over days) or insidiously (over months) [Bohan and Peters, 1975; Dalakas, 1991; Griggs et al., 1995; Amato et al., 1996; Amato and Barohn, 1997]. The earliest and most severely affected muscle groups are the neck flexor, shoulder girdle, and pelvic girdle muscles. Inflammation of oropharyngeal and esophageal muscles leads to dysphagia in approximately 30% of the DM patients [Bohan and Peters, 1975; Dalakas, 1991; Engel et al., 1994; Griggs et al., 1995].

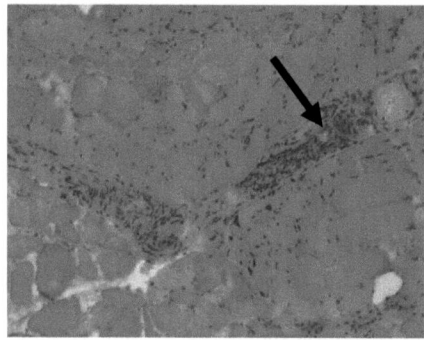

Figure 9: *Dermatomyositis: hematoxylin and eosin (H&E) paraffin section. In dermatomyositis, the characteristic inflammation is perivascular within the perimysial connective tissue. In this image, a perivascular lymphocytic infiltrate is associated with a blood vessel, indicated by the arrow. A few red blood cells within the lumen assist in identifying this as a blood vessel. The surrounding myofibers and endomysium are not inflamed.*

Early recognition and diagnosis of DM is facilitated because of the characteristic rash that may accompany or precede the onset of muscle weakness [Dalakas et al., 1991; Engel at al., 1994; Griggs et al., 1995; Amato and Barohn, 1997]. The classic skin manifestations include a heliotrope rash (purplish discoloration of the eyelids often associated with periorbital edema) and Gottron sign (popular, erythematous, scaly lesions over the knuckles): in addition, a flat, erythematous, sun-sensitive rash may appear on the face, neck, and anterior chest (V-sign); on the shoulders and upper back (shawl sign); and on the elbows, knees, and malleoli.

Characteristic features of DM: Serum CK is the most sensitive and specific marker of muscle destruction and is elevated in more than 90% of DM patients [Amato et al., 1996; Amato and Barohn, 1997]. Serum CK levels can be normal or as high as 50 times the normal value. However, serum CK levels do not directly correlate with the severity of weakness and can be normal even in markedly weak individuals, particularly in childhood DM [Dalakas, 1991; Griggs et al., 1995; Pachman, 1995].

Perifascicular atrophy is the characteristic histological feature, occurring in as many as 90% of children and in at least 50% of adults with DM [Dalakas, 1991; Engel at al., 1994; Amato and Barohn, 1997; Amato and Shebert, 1998]. The perifascicular area contains small degenerating fibres and atrophic and non-atrophic fibres with microvaculation and disrupted oxidative enzyme staining. Occasionally, microinfarcts of muscle fascicles are apparent. Scattered necrotic fibres may be present;

however, in contrast to PM and IBM, invasion of non-necrotic fibres is not seen. Inflammation, when present, is predominantly perivascular and located in the perimysium rather than the endomysium. Electron microscopy reveals small intramuscular blood vessels (arterioles and capillaries) with endothelial hyperplasia, microvacoules, and cytoplasmic inclusions; these abnormalities precede other structural abnormalities in electron microscopy [Banker, 1975; DeVisser, 1989]. DM can also occur as paraneoplastic disease. In absence of malignancy, prognosis is favourable in patients with DM.

1.7.2 Polymyositis

PM generally presents in patients older than age 20 years. Similar to DM, it is more prevalent in women [Medgser et al., 1970; Bohan and Peters, 1975; Tymms and Webb, 1985; Dalakas, 1991; Engel et al., 1994; Griggs et al., 1995; Amato et al., 1996; Amato and Barohn, 1997]. Compared with DM, there is often a delay from onset of symptoms to diagnosis, perhaps there is no associated rash, which serves as a red flag to patients and their physicians. As with DM, patients typically present with neck flexor and symmetric proximal arm and leg weakness developing over several weeks or months [Bohan and Peters, 1975; Amato et al., 1996]. Distal muscles may also become involved but are not as weak as the proximal muscles [Griggs et al., 1995; Amato et al., 1996]. Myalgias and tenderness are common. Dysphagia occurs in approximately one-third of patients secondary to oropharyngeal and esophageal involvements [Tymms and Webb, 1985; Dalakas, 1991;

Engel et al., 1994; Griggs et al., 1995]. Sensation and muscle stretch reflexes are usually normal.

Characteristic features: Serum CK level is elevated 5- to 50-folds in the majority of PM cases [Tymms and Webb, 1985; Dalakas, 1991; Engel et al., 1994; Griggs et al., 1995; Amato et al., 1996; Amato and Barohn, 1997]. As in DM, serum CK levels can be elevated in patients who have normal manual muscle function testing, whereas weak patients can have normal levels. Muscle biopsies are characterized by variability in fibre size, scattered necrotic and regenerating fibres, and endomysial inflammation with invasion of nonnecrotic muscle fibres. The endomysial inflammatory cells consist primarily of activated CD8+ (cytotoxic), alpha, beta T cells, and macrophages [Arahata and Engel, 1984; Engel and Arahata, 1984; Engel et al., 1994]. PM can develop in patients infected with HIV and human T-lymphocyte virus-1 (HTLV-1) [Dalakas, 1991; Amato and Barohn, 1997]. The myositis associated with HIV and HTLV-1 infections appears to be result of indirect triggering of the immune response against muscle fibres. Most patients with PM improve with immunosuppressive therapies, although many require lifelong treatment [Tymms and Webb, 1985; DeVisser et al., 1989; Chwalinska-Sadowska and Madykova, 1990].

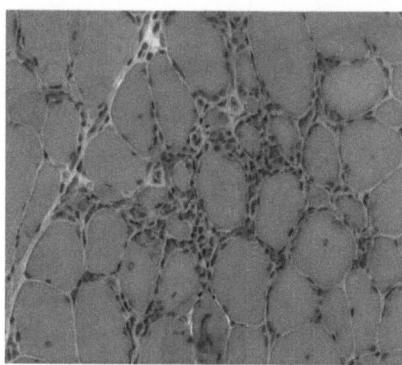

Figure 10: Polymyositis: hematoxylin and eosin (H&E) frozen section. The numerous small dark blue cells constitute a dense, chronic, endomysial lymphocytic inflammatory infiltrate. This section also shows many rounded atrophic myofibers, an increase in internal nuclei, and moderate endomysial fibrosis.

1.7.3 Inclusion body myositis

Sporadic IBM presents with an insidious onset of slowly progressive proximal and distal weakness [Dalakas, 1991; Amato et al., 1996; Amato and Barohn, 1997; Griggs et al., 1995]. Although IBM is the most common inflammatory myopathy in patients older than age 50 years, it is frequently misdiagnosed. The slow evolution of the disease process probably accounts in part for the delay in diagnosis, averaging approximately 6 years from onset of symptoms [Lotz et al., 1989; Amato et al., 1996]. Unlike the female predominance seen with DM and PM, men are much more commonly affected than women in IBM. In addition, IBM patients have a unique pattern of weakness, with early weakness and atrophy of the quadriceps, volar forearm muscle (i.e., wrist and fingerflexor), and ankle dorsiflexors [Lotz et al., 1989; Amato et al., 1996]. As many as 40% of the patients report dysphagia, which can be so severe that some patients require cricopharyngeal myotomy [Lotz et al., 1989; Darrow et al., 1992]. Approximately one-third of the IBM patients have mild facial weakness [Lotz et al., 1989; Amato et al., 1996]. There are hereditary forms of inclusion body *myopathy*, but these are clinically and histologically distinct from the more common sporadic inclusion body *myositis*. Hereditary autosomal recessive inclusion body myopathy has no inflammations on muscle biopsy and spares the quadriceps muscle [Argov and Yarom, 1984].

Characteristic features: Unlike DM and PM, the serum CK is normal or only mildly elevated (less than 10-folds above normal) in patients with IBM [Askanas et al., 1993; Amato et al., 1996]. Muscle biopsies characteristically demonstrate endomysial inflammation, small groups of atrophic fibres, eosinophilic cytoplasmic inclusions, and muscle fibres with one or more rimmed vacuoles lined with granular material [Lotz et al., 1989]. Amyloid deposition is evident on Congo red staining using polarized light or fluorescence technique [Askanas et al., 1993]. Electron microscopy demonstrates 15- to 21-nm cytoplasmic and intranuclear tubulofilaments [Lotz et al., 1989]. In addition, 6- to 10-nm tubulofilaments can also be found in the cytoplasm of vacuolated muscle fibres [Griggs et al 1995 (b)]. The endomysial inflammation in IBM is composed of macrophages and CD8+ cytotoxic/suppressor T lymphocytes that invade non-necrotic fibres, like in PM [Engel and Arahata, 1984; Mikol et al., 1994; Griggs et al. 1995 b].

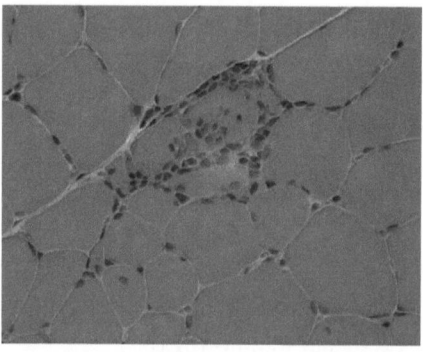

Figure 11: *Inclusion body myositis: eosinophilic inclusion on hematoxylin and eosin (H&E) frozen section. The myofibers in the central region of the image contain dense eosinophilic inclusions surrounded by basophilic granular material. These inclusions may be cytoplasmic, within rimmed vacuoles, or they may be present within nuclei. These inclusions label for amyloid precursor protein, ubiquitin, tau, and prion protein, which are characteristic of central neurodegenerative diseases.*

The pathogenesis of IBM is unknown. IBM may be primary inflammatory myopathy like DM and PM. However, a primary degenerative myopathic disorder, such as a dystrophy with secondary inflammation, is also a possibility [Griggs et al 1995 b].
Patients with IBM do not significantly improve with immunosuppressive treatment [Dalakas, 1991; Mikol et al., 1994; Griggs et al., 1995; Amato

and Barohn, 1997]. Life expectancy does not appear to be significantly altered. Most patients remain ambulatory, although they frequently require a cane or a wheelchair for long-distance movements. However, some patients become severely incapacitated and require a wheelchair within 10-15 years [Lotz et al., 1989]. A recent pilot study conducted with 13 sIBM patients showed that infusion of a humanized monoclonal antibody Alemtuzumab can slow down disease progression and reduces endomysial inflammation and stressor molecules [Dalakas et al., 2009].

Table 1: Idiopathic inflammatory myopathies: clinical and laboratory features [Amato and Barohn, 1997]

	Sex	Typical age at onset	Rash	Patterns of weakness	CK	Muscle biopsy	Cellular infiltrate	Response to immuno-supressive therapy	Common associated conditions
DM	Female > male	Childhood and adult	yes	Proximal > distal	Increased (up to 50X)	Perimysial and perivascular inflammation; membrane attack complex, immuno-globulin, complement deposition on vessels	CD4+ cells; B cells	Yes	Myocarditis, interstitial lung disease, malignancy, vasculitis, other connective tissue diseases
PM	Female > male	Adult	No	Proximal > distal	Increased (up to 50X)	Endomysial inflammation	CD8+ T cells; Macro-phages	Yes	Myocarditis, interstitial lung disease, other connective tissue diseases
IBM	Male > female	Elderly (>50 yrs.)	No	Proximal = distal; predilection for finger/wrist flexors and knee extensors	Normal or mildly increased (< 10X)	Endomysial inflammation; rimmed vacuoles; amyloid deposits; electron microscopy: 15- to 18- nm tubulo-filaments	CD8+ T cells; Macro-phages	None or minimal	Neuropathy, autoimmune disorders - uncommon

2. Background of the study

Mitochondrial abnormalities in sIBM were identified and described as early as in 1975 [Carpenter et al., 1975]. Studies reported that the morphological changes such as muscle fibres with abnormal proliferation, some of them being ragged-red fibres and fibres with deficiency of enzyme-histochemical COX activity are frequent in sIBM but can also be observed in DM and PM [Rifai et al., 1995; Oldfors et al., 1995].

Several studies reported mitochondrial abnormalities in inflammatory myopathies. In one series, COX-deficient fibres were not observed in inflammatory myopathies [Yamamoto et al., 1989], in another, COX deficiency was mostly limited to necrotic fibres [Doriguzzi et al., 1990]. However, the age of the patients and the nature of the underlying neuromuscular disease (PM vs DM vs IBM) were not evaluated in these studies. Other investigations seem to report mild mitochondrial abnormalities (COX-deficient fibres) in DM (0.8%) and PM (0.2%) compared to an age-matched group [Chariot et al., 1996]. Another study that evaluated 10 patients with diagnosis of DM and 15 age and gender matched healthy individuals reported an increased percentage of COX-negative and SDH hyper-reactive fibres in DM patients (0.82% and 1.82% respectively) compared to controls (0.26% and 0.22% respectively) [Miro et al., 1998]. Similarly, one another study reports abnormal COX and SDH histochemical activities in atrophic perifascicular fibres being the characteristic features of DM [Alhatou et al., 2004]. Furthermore, studies suggest that mitochondrial changes are more common in IBM than in PM. MtDNA deletions have been found in at least half of patient population with IBM by *in situ* hybridization [Oldfors et al., 1993; Oldfors et al., 1995] and PCR analysis [Oldfors et al., 1995]. The mitochondrial abnormalities in IBM are manifest by an excess of muscle fibres with deficient COX activity and ragged-red fibres with excessive staining for succinate dehydrogenase (SDH) [Oldfors et al., 1993]. Histological and biochemical mitochondrial abnormalities have also been described in PM [Watkins and Cullen, 1987; Campos et al., 1995], but are generally thought to be unusual [Rifai et al., 1995].

In addition to histological and biochemical mitochodrial abnormalities, mtDNA changes are also frequently identified in myositis. Multiple deletions are detected in the DNA of patients with different types of myositis but the frequency and the degrees of deletions and their correlation with histological features and the biochemical enzyme activity have not yet been reported.

2.1 Inclusion body myositis and mtDNA deletions

Multiple mtDNA deletions have been identified in most of the IBM patients by using sensitive PCR analysis [Rötig et al., 1992; Bua et al., 2006]. Interestingly, the more quantitative Southern-blot analysis seems to fails in demonstrating the deletions in more than half of the patients [Samuel et al., 2004; Bender et al., 2006; Bua et al., 2006] due to lower sensitivity of the method. This findings suggest that the amount of mtDNA with deletions is very much variable and in most of the cases it is very low. Numerous deletions were identified in patients with IBM, the 4977 bp deletion being most frequent. Oldfors et al report that the common 4977 bp deletion (CD) was identified in very high levels (>90%) in 9 out of 60 fibres from four different patients with IBM [Oldfors et al., 2006]. Moreover, many of the deletions identified were not flanked by direct repeats. All the mutations were spread through the ND4 region.

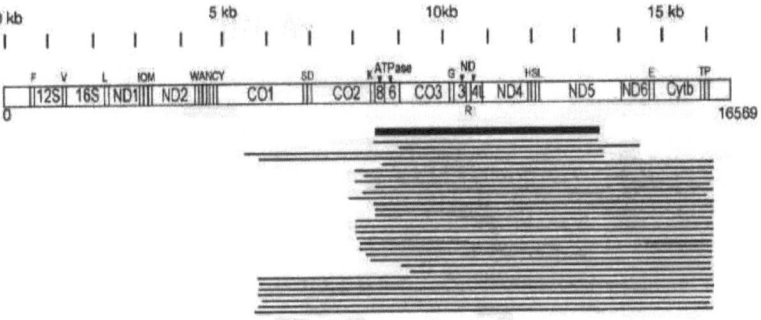

Figure 12: Distribution of 32 different mtDNA deletions in IBM patient, the common 4977 bp deletion (CD) is shown by bold line [Oldfors et al., 2006].

In IBM, the clonal expansion of the CD has been found to be a frequent cause of COX deficient fibres and some COX deficient fibres are also probably due to clonal expansion of point mutation [Oldfors et al., 2006].

2.2 Polymyositis/dermatomyositis and mtDNA deletions

MtDNA deletions are also reported in two cases with PM (Molnar and Schröder, 1998). In one of the two PM cases, a single large deletion between the nucleotides 9990 and 11450 was found while the other showed multiple mtDNA deletions in positions 3000-4500 and 8340-11450. The presence of mtDNA deletions in muscle fibres of patients with DM is not published so far.

Since no single detailed study comparing the genetic, biochemical and histological features in patients with different forms of myositis, the current study is aimed towards the analysis of mitochondrial DNA deletions in patients with different forms of myositis and to identify a possible correlation (if any) between frequency of mtDNA deletions and biochemical and histological abnormalities.

3. Patients

The study included three groups of myositis patients and a control group.

3.1 Myositis patients

The patients were grouped into three definite groups of myositis on the basis of following criteria.

13 of the DM patients (n=14; male: 6, female: 8; Age: 37-84 yrs., Mean: 61 yrs.) fulfilled the **Bohan and Peter's criteria** [Bohan and Peters, 1975] for definite dermatomyositis and 1 patient fulfilled the possible criteria.

8 of the PM patients (n=12; male: 6, female: 6; Age: 33-77 yrs., Mean: 62 yrs.) fulfilled the Bohan and Peter's [Bohan and Peters, 1975] criteria for definite polymyositis and four patients fulfilled the criteria of probable polymyositis.

All the IBM patients (n=9; male: 5, female: 4; Age: 57-72 yrs., Mean: 64 yrs.) fulfilled the definite criteria according to Griggs [Griggs et al., 1995 b].

Bohan and Peter's criteria PM/DM

1. Symmetrical weakness, usually progressive, of the limb-girdle muscles.

2. Muscle biopsy evidence of myositis:
- Necrosis of type I and type II muscle fibers, Phagocytosis, Degeneration and regeneration of myofibers with variation in myofiber size, Endomysial, perimysial, perivascular or interstitial mononuclear cells.

3. Elevation of serum levels of muscle-associated enzymes:

- CK, Aldolase, LDH, Transaminases (ALT/ and AST).

4. Electromyographic triad of myopathy:

- Short, small, low-amplitude polyphasic motor unit potentials.
- Fibrillation potentials, even at rest.
- Bizarre high-frequency repetitive discharges.

5. Characteristic rashes of dermatomyositis:

Definite PM=all first 4, probable PM=3 of first 4, possible PM=2 of 4;

Definite DM= rash + 3 other; probable DM=rash + 2 other; possible DM=rash + 1 other

Griggs' criteria for IBM

A. Clinical Features:

1. Duration > 6 mos.
2. Age of onset > 30 yrs.
3. Pattern of Weaknes:

a. Finger flexor weakness.

b. Wrist flexor > wrist extensor weakness.

c. Quadriceps weakness (= or < MRC grade 4).

B. Laboratory Features:

1. Serum CK < 12 x normal.
2. Muscle biopsy:

a. mononuclear inflammatory cells invasion of non-necrotic muscle fibers.

b. vacuolated muscle fibers.

c. either,

i. intracellulat amyloid deposits.

ii. 15-18 nm tubulofilaments by EM.

3. EMG

a. ''features of an inflammatory myopathy''.

b. May have long-duration MUAPs.

Definite IBM

- Patient must exhibit all muscle biopsy features.

- None of the clinical or other laboratory features are required if patient meets Bx criteria.

Possible IBM

- Bx shows only inflammation and invasion of fibers without vacuoles, amyloid, or TF on EM.

- Meets all Clinical Criteria (1,2,3) and other lab criteria (1,3)

3.2 Normal controls

The group contained normal controls (n=10). DNA was extracted from patients with myalgia who underwent diagnostic biopsies but after detailed clinical investigations, a neuromuscular disorder was not identified. The CK- value was not increased (< 2,8 µmol/ls) (range: 0,63-2,44), EMG was normal and myohistologically the patients had no indication of myopathy. The patients had no muscle weakness. Six females and four males were included in the study and the age ranged from 45 to 69 years with mean age of 53 years.

4. Materials and methods

4.1 Materials
4.1.1 DNA extraction
DNA extraction kit: PeqGOLD DNA kit (PeQLab biotechnologies), Absolute alcohol, Proteinase K

4.1.2 Long-range PCR
PCR Primers (Invitrogen), Enzyme mix (Expanded long PCR system from Roche), dNTP mix, BSA, Buffer 3, Agarose powder (UltraPure from Invitrogen life technologies), Ethidium bromide, DNA Marker X (Roche), Gel analysis software: gene tools, version 3.03(b) (Syngene, Synoptics Ltd, USA)

4.1.3 Common deletion PCR
PCR primers (Invitrogen), PCR buffer, dNTP mix, $MgCl_2$, Taq Polymerase, Agarose powder (UltraPure from Invitrogen life technologies), Ethidium bromide, DNA Marker 100 (Fermentas)

4.1.4 Southern Blot
Restriction enzyme BamHI, Restriction enzyme ApaI, Agarose powder (UltraPure from Invitrogen life technologies), Nitrocellulose membrane, 16-s and 18-s DIG labelled DNA probes with PCR DIG DNA probe synthesis kit (Roche), DIG marked markers X and II (Roche), ECL-kit (Biological Industries Ltd.)

4.1.5 Real-time PCR

PCR primers: common deletion and HVR2 region (Invitrogen), FastStart Universal SYBR Green Master (ROX) kit (Roche), Plasmid (PCR.Script Amp (SK+) vector in XI-1 blue cells (Stratagene, USA), Thermocycler: Rotor-Gene (Corbett Research), Real-time analysis software: Rotor-Gene (Corbett Research)

4.1.6 Multiple-cell PCR

Microtome (Leica microsystems), Incubation medium, Sodium Phosphate buffer pH 7.4, SDH solution, Alcohol (different concentrations), Xylol, Micro-laser dissector (PALM® Microbeam (P.A.L.M) microlaser tech. USA), Elution buffer (PeQLab biotechnologies), Proteinase K, Materials required for Real-time PCR

4.1.7 Biochemical COX /CS activity

Ultra pure water (Biochrom AG), Enzyme diluting buffer, Detergent (n-Dodecyl ß-D-Maltosid), Homogenizing buffer, Assay Buffer, Dimethiothreitol (DTT) (Aldrich), Cytochrome C (Sigma)

4.2 Methods

For quantitative and qualitative analysis of mitochondrial DNA, whole DNA was extracted from muscles homogenate of all the controls and patients.

4.2.1 Extraction of DNA from muscle

DNA was extracted from muscle using *peqGOLD Tissue DNA mini kit*:
   1- 30 mg of muscle tissue was cut in a clean 1.5 ml centrifuge tube.

2- 200 µl TL-buffer and 25 µl Protease were added in the tube and vortexed. The mixture was incubated at 55°C for 3 hours. The mixture was vortexed every 20-30 minutes.

3- After 3 hours of incubation 200 µl BL-buffer was added in the tube and vortexed. The mixture was incubated at 70°C for 10 minutes.

4- 220 µl of absolute alcohol was added in the tube and vortexed to mix the solution homogenously. The DNA column (provided with the kit) was placed over 2 ml collecting tube and up to 650 µl of the mixture was transferred over the column. Centrifuged at 8000 rpm for 1 minute. Centrifuged again until all the liquid is used up.

5- The column was again placed over new collecting tube and 600 µl of washing buffer was added to it and centrifuged at 8000 rpm for 1 minute.

6- Step 5 was repeated.

7- The column was placed over new collecting tube and centrifuged at full speed for 2 minutes for complete drying of the DNA.

8- The column was placed over new centrifuge tube and 200µl of pre warmed (70°C) elution buffer was added over it and incubated at room temperature for 3 minutes and then centrifuged at 8000 rpm for 1 minute.

9- Elution step 8 was repeated and the DNA was collected in collection tubes.

10- The concentration of the extracted DNA was measured by spectralphotometric method, measuring the absorption of 1:25 diluted (in Aqua bidest) DNA at 260 and 280 nm.

4.2.2 Qualitative analysis: mtDNA deletions

Qualitative analysis included the analysis of mtDNA using following protocols:
- Long-range PCR
- Common deletion PCR
- Southern-blot

4.2.2.1 Long-range-PCR

Identification of thermostable DNA polymerase for routine laboratory diagnostics in the year 1994 [Cheng et al., 1994; Barnes, 1994] made amplication of DNA molecule, rather, quite easy and convenient. The long-range PCR employed in this study is a slightly modified PCR technique than the normal PCR. Unlike the normal PCR which is used to amplify shorter fragments of DNA, long-range PCR contains the PCR mix that is able to amplify rather larger fragments and as the name itself suggests is run for a longer time. The Expanded Long Template PCR system (Roche) contains a unique enzyme mix with thermostable Taq DNA polymerase and Tgo DNA polymerase, a thermostable DNA polymerase with proofreading activity. The powerful polymerase mixture produces a high yield of PCR products from genomic DNA.

4.2.2.1.1 Modification of long-range-PCR

To increase the sensitivity of the deletions with various lengths, few modifications in the normal long-range PCR reaction were done.
- Modification of elongation time: The elongation time was determined with respect to the length of the amplified DNA

fragments, ie, bigger the fragment, longer the elongation time and vice-versa. It is therefore expected that a smaller (deleted) mtDNA fragment at shorter (than in the standard conditions) elongation time is preferred (instead of the longer wild-type fragment) is amplified (Luoma et al., 2005). For a better representation of the singular mtDNA deletions in the 10kb-PCR, three different elongations times of 10 minutes (standard conditions), 4 - and 2 minutes were applied. The repetition of elongation time should take place by 20 seconds from the 11th cycle.

- Modification of DNA concentration and dNTPs in PCR mix: The DNA concentration and concentration of the dNTPs were calculated by hit and trial method, retaining the best and the optimal concentration.

The PCR primers were so designed that the primers incorporate 10 kb fragment of the mtDNA in the major arc region where almost all the deletions are found to be located.

Long-range PCR process also comprises of three steps (denatuturatiuon, hybridization, and elongation) which are continuously repeated in a thermocycler [Mullis and Faloona, 1987].

Primers:

Primer:	mt-Position	5' Sequence-3'
Long 10 kb-F	6221-6239	CCCTCTCTCCTACTCCTG
Long 10 kb-R	16153-16133	CAGGTGGTCAAGTATTTATGG

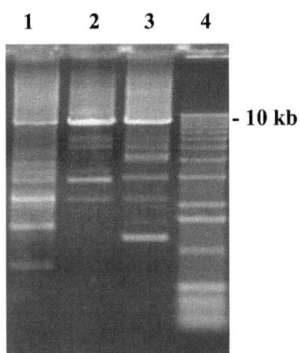

Figure 13: Multiple deletions in Long-range PCR with prominent 10 kb wild type band in all the samples (lanes 1, 2, and 3) follwed by marker in lane 4.

PCR Protocol:

Mastermix 1

1.5 µl Primer 10kb-F (10pmol/l)

1.5 µl Primer 10kb-R (10pmol/l)

2.5 µl dNTP-Mix

18.5 µl H_2O

Mastermix 2

10 µl BSA 0,1%

5 µl Buffer 3 (27,5 mM $MgCl_2$ und Tenside)

8.55 µl H_2O

0.45 µl Enzyme-Mix (Expanded Long Template Enzyme Mix Roche 1U in 5 µl)

DNA-Volume: 2 µl

Temperature Profile:

	Denaturation	10 Cycles			20 Cycles			Final Elongation	
Temp. (°C)	93	93	57	68	93	57	68	68	4
Time (Min.)	3:00	0:30	0:30	10:00	0:30	0:30	10:0-16:20	10:0	∞

The large PCR products were separated on 0.8% agarose gel.

4.2.2.2 Common deletion PCR

The PCR is designed to detect a particular sequence in the mtDNA which encompasses the 4977 bp common deletion (CD). The CD is flanked by a 13 bp direct repeat, the 5' end starting at nucleotide position 8469 in ND4 region and ending at nucleotide position 13446. The primers are so designed that they bind at the either side of the region of CD. If the deletion is persistent in the template, the PCR will amplify a DNA fragment of 470 bp excluding the 4977 bp that the CD encompasses. If there is no deletion, the fragment to be amplified would be a very large fragment (470+4977 bp) which will not be amplified by this normal PCR protocol.

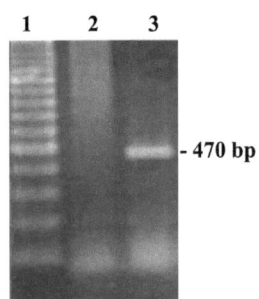

Figure 14: Common deletion PCR with 477 bp band (lane 3). First lane is 100 bp marker followed by CD negative sample in lane 2 and CD positive sample in lane 3.

Primers:

Primer:	mt-Position	5' Sequence-3'
CD-F	8274-8305	CCCTCTACCCCCTCTAGAGCCCACTGTAAA GC
CD-R	13720-13692	GGCTTCCGGCTGCCAGGCCTTTAATGGGG

PCR Protocol:

Mastermix

2.5 µl Primer CD-F (10pmol/l)

2.5 µl Primer CD-R (10pmol/l)

2.5 µl PCR-Buffer II

0.5 µl dNTP-Mix

1.5 µl MgCl$_2$

13.3 µl H$_2$O

0,2 µl Taq-Polymerase: 0.2 µl

DNA-Volume: 2 µl

Temperature profile:

	Denaturation	32 Cycles			Final Elongation	
Temp. (°C)	94	94	70	72	72	4
Time (Min.)	1:0	1:0	0:30	1:0	10:0	∞

Electrophoresis was done on 2% agarose gel.

4.2.2.3 Southern-blot analysis

Southern-blot analysis was performed as described previously [Sambrook and Russel, 2001] in 9 patients with myositis and in 9 patients with CPEO (that have higher degree of heteroplasmy of the common deletion) as positive controls to compare results of the real-time PCR analysis (described separately below). The method is based on the digestion of the DNA with a specific restriction enzyme that cuts the circular mtDNA once. For this method restriction endonuclese BamHI was used and separation of the resulting fragments was done by electrophoresis that was performed on 0.8% agarose gel at 30 V for overnight

The double stranded DNA fragment is separated to single stands through an alkaline buffer and finally transferred to nitrocellulose membrane and heat fixed. Hybridization (attachment of the single-strand DNA fragment to the complementary DNA) was done at 50°C for 12-16 hours.

The primer sequences for preparation of DNA probe using Long-Range-

PCR were as following:

16-s rRNA Sense: AAG CGT TCA AGC TCA ACA CC
Antisense: CTA CCT TTG CAC GGT TAG GG

A 15 kb fragment was amplified covering nearly the whole mitochondrial genome. This fragment was cut with ApaI in 5 pieces before hybridization. 16-s and 18-s DIG labelled DNA probes with PCR DIG DNA probe synthesis kit from Roche and DIG marked markers X and II (Roche) with DIG DNA labelling kit from Roche were prepared. The film was developed on ECL-kit (Biological Industries Ltd.)

4.2.3 Quantitative analysis: mtDNA common deletion

In order to quantify the level of common deletion in patients in three groups of myositis and controls in the study, a quantitative real-time PCR method was employed.

4.2.3.1 Real-time PCR analysis

Standard PCR method is limited mainly to qualitative analysis of the DNA. With time the technical effort involved in standard PCR got directed more toward positive recognition of the amplicons. The important methods of post-PCR analysis rely on either size or sequence of the amplicon. Gel electrophoresis is often used to measure the size of the amplicon and this is both inexpensive and simple to implement. Unfortunately, size analysis has limited specificity since different molecules of approximately the same molecular weight can not be distinguished. Consequently, gel electrophoresis alone is not a sufficient PCR end-point in many instances, including most clinical applications. Characterization of the product by its sequence is far more reliable and informative. Probe hybridisation assays for this purpose are available but many are multi-step procedures. Such methods are time-consuming and care must be taken to ensure that amplicons accidently released into the laboratory environment do not contaminate the DNA preparations and clean rooms.

Real-time PCR method allows the quantitative analysis of the amplicons on the basis of fluorescent signals obtained. There are two general approaches used to obtain fluorescent signal from the synthesis of product in PCR. The first depends upon the property of fluorescent dyes such as SYBR green I to bind to double stranded DNA and undergo a conformational change that result in an increase in their fluorescence. The second approach is to use fluorescence resonance energy transfer (FRET). These methods use a variety of means to alter the relative spatial arrangement of photon donor and acceptor molecules. These molecules are attached to probes, primers or the PCR product and are usually selected to that amplification of a specific DNA sequence brings about an increase in fluorescence at a particular wavelength.

The real-time PCR instrumentations and signal transduction system allows to characterize the PCR amplicon *in situ* on the machine. This is done by analysis of the melting temperature and/or probe hybridization characteristics of the amplicon within the PCR reaction mixture. In the intercalating dye system the melting temperature of the amplicon can be estimated by measuring the level of fluorescence emitted by the dye as the temperature is increased from below to above the expected melting temperature. The methods that rely upon probe hybridisation to produce a fluorescent signal are generally less liable to produce false positive results than alternative methods such as the use of intercalating dyes to detect net synthesis of double stranded DNA followed by melting analysis of the product. Hybridisation, ResonSence and hydrolysis probe system give fluorescent signals that are only produced when the target sequence is amplified and are unlikely to give false positive results. An additional feature of hybridisation, ResonSence and related methods is that it is also possible to measure the temperature at which the probes disassociate from their complementary sequences giving further verification of the specificity of the amplification reaction. An important feature of many probe systems is that they are compatible with resolvable emission spectra.

4.2.3.1.1 Implementation of real-time PCR analysis in present study

To quantify the degree of common deletion (CD), quantitative real-time PCR was designed with an 350 bp amplicon measuring the CD and the 400 bp reference sequence of the hypervariable region 2 (HVR2) found in the mitochondrial D-loop. This HVR2 segment was taken as a reference fragment, since it contains essential elements which are not affected by deletions in replicating mitochondrial DNA molecules. Hence, it represents the total amount of mtDNA in a tissue sample. Primer sequences for the 350 bp CD amplicon and HVR2-region were designed as previously described [Sabunciyan et al., 2007].

Common deletion:

Forward: CCC CTC TAG AGC CCA CTG TA

Reverse: GAG TGC TAT AGG GGC TTG TC

HVR2-region:

Forward: CTC TCA CCC TAT TAA CCA CT

Reverse: GTT AAA AGT GCA TAC CGC CA

All SYBR green reactions were carried out in Rotor-Gene (Corbett Research) cycler using FastStart Universal SYBR Green Master (ROX) kit (Roche).

The temperature profile:

Hold 1@ 93°C for 3 min.

Cycling (40 repeats) Step 1 @ 93°C, hold 60 sec.

Step 2 @ 56°C, hold 40 sec.

Step 3 @ 72°C, hold 60 sec.

Step 4 @ 79°C, hold 20°C, acquiring to cycling A (Sybr).

Hold 2 @ 72°C for 7 min

Melt (72-79°C) hold 5 sec, acquiring to melt A (Sybr).

Dilution series of plasmids containing CD break point and the HVR-2 region were used to calibrate the quantification by Rotor-Gene real-time analysis software. The plasmids were received from Dr. Kirches, Dept. of Neuropathology Magdeburg. The primers were used as described previously [Sabunciyan et al., 2007]. They were constructed from DNA of a patient with 50% CD in skeletal muscle and blood samples (HVR2), using the PCR.Script Amp (SK+) vector in XI-1 blue cells (Stratagene, USA). Both dilution series spanned a range of 10000-folds dilution in four decadic steps, resulting in standard curves of high linearity (r>0.98). A melting profile was automatically generated after 40 PCR cycles, by slowly melting the double stranded DNA. A single peak was visible in the plot dF/dT versus T (velocity of fluorescence versus temperature) for plasmid and DNA samples for both amplified regions. The peak was not present in controls containing only PCR premix without template DNA.

4.2.4 Control of real-time PCR protocol

Since the degree of CD in patients with idiopathic myositis is very low, the result obtained by using real time-PCR needs to be as précised as possible. As Southern-blot was not able to detect such a low degree of heteroplasmy, the real-time PCR protocol lacks from the benefit of control that could be used to check the results. In order to believe and accept the degree of heteroplasmy of the CD in patients with myositis, obtained by real-time PCR, the real time PCR protocol needed to be controlled with the help of CPEO patients with known degree of the CD. For this, real-time PCR analysis of CPEO patients (n=9) to identify the degree of heteroplasmy of the CD was done as described above. Simultaneously, the Southern-blot analysis of DNA of the same patients was also done as described above. The degree of heteroplysmy of the CD was calculated by using the gel analysis software, Gene Tools, version 3.03(b) (Syngene, Synoptics Ltd, USA). The efficiency of the real-time PCR analysis was known by comparing the degrees of heteroplasmy of the CD obtained by both the methods.

4.2.5 Multiple-cell real-time PCR

The normal real-time PCR analysis of whole DNA gives the approximate heteroplasmy level in the muscle homeogenate as the DNA mixture contains DNA from both normal- and COX deficient cells. In order to make the finding more specific and accurate, real-time PCR analysis using the DNA extracted from 10 individual normal and COX deficient cells each from biopsy samples was performed. Following steps were followed for multiple-cell real-time PCR analysis.

4.2.5.1 COX/SDH staining:

1. 10 µm thin cryo- cross sections of the biopsy were cut under microtome
2. The sections were covered with 50 µl of the incubation medium on a glass slide.
3. The slide was incubated at 37°C for 60 min.
4. Slide was washed with 0.05 M sodium phosphate buffer pH 7.4
5. The section over the slide was covered with 50 µl of SDH solution.
6. The slide was incubated at 37°C for 60 min.
7. The slide was washed with aquadest and incorporated to alcohol series as following:

70% alcohol	a while
96% alcohol	30 sec.
absolute alcohol (2X)	2 min. each
Xylol (2X)	2 min. each

4.2.5.2 Dissection of single cells and DNA extraction:

1. 10 individual normal (brown stained) and 10 COX deficient (blue stained) fibres were dissected in separate collecting tubes under

PALM ® MicroBeam, micro laser dissector (P.A.L.M. microlaser technologies, USA).

2. To the tubes containing muscle fibres, 10 µl of elution buffer from PeqGOLD DNA kit (PeQLab biotechnologies) and 4 µl of 10% proteinase K were added and mixed well.
3. The tubes were incubated at 55°C for 1 hour.
4. The remaining enzyme was heat deactivated at 95°C for 10 minutes.
5. The DNA in the tubes was stored at 4°C for further use.
6. Real-time PCR was performed using the DNA extracted from individual normal and COX deficient fibres as described above.

4.2.6 Biochemical enzyme activity

Cytrate synthase (CS) and cytochrome c oxidase (COX) activities were measured in all the controls and myositis patients using standard photometric methods.

4.2.6.1 Citrate synthase activity

Citrate synthase is assayed by measuring the rate of production of coenzyme A (CoA.SH) from oxaloacetate by measuring free sulfhydryl groups using the thiol reagent 5,5'-dithio-bis-(2-nitobenzoic acid) (DTNB). DTNB reacts spontaneously with sulfhydryl groups to produce free 5-thio-2-nitrobenzoate anions, which have a yellow colour and can be monitored at 412nm.

Principle of the assay:

Acetyl-CoA + Oxalacetat ⟶ Citrate + CoA-SH ⟶ CoA-SH + DTNB ⟶ CoA-DTNB

Bovine muscle homogenate was diluted to 1:1000 in Chappel-Perry medium. 10 µL of the
homogenate was added in a cuvette containing Tris Mannitol (900 µL), 5% Triton (20 µL), DTNB (10 µL), Acetyl-Co A (50 µL). The reaction was incubated at 30°C for 10 minutes followed by addition of 10 µL of Oxalacetate.
Absorption was measured at 412nm for 220 sec. CS activity was then mathematically calculated.

4.2.6.2 COX activity

Muscle homogenate was prepared (concentration 1:30) by diluting the muscle in enzyme diluting buffer and 1mM Detergent (n-Dodecyl ß-D-Maltosid). The homogenate was left in the homoginator over ice for 5-7 minutes. The homogenate was centrifuged at 2500 rpm (U/min) at 25°C in Eppendorf centrifuge 5415R. Bovine muscle (1:10 in liquid nitrogen) was taken as control. The absorption of Cyt c was measured at a wavelength of 550nm. The extinction coefficient at 550nm is 21.84. The measurement of the absorption was done for first 45 seconds reaction. The total volume of the reaction solution was 1.1 mL.
For protein residue: 20 µL Homogenate (1:30) in 180 µL 50 mM NaOH was taken.

For residual citrate synthase, 30 µL Homogenate (1:30) in 69 µL Assay buffer was taken.

The activitity of COX was then mathematically calculated. The ratio of activities of COX and CS activities was expresses as residual enzyme in percentage.

5. Results

5.1 Molecular genetic findings:

5.1.1 Long-range PCR

In the control group, two subjects (20%) were found to harbour multiple deletions.

In the dermatomyositis group, seven (54%) patients were found to harbour multiple deletions.

In the polymyositis group, five patients (42%) were found to harbour multiple deletions.

In the IBM group, all patients (100%) were found to harbour both multiple deletions.

Individual results of the patients are shown in table 2 column 2.

5.1.2 Common deletion PCR :

In the control group, two subjects (20%) were found to the common deletion.

In the dermatomyositis, group five (38%) patients were found to harbour the common deletion, respectively.

In the polymyositis group, five patients (42%) were found to harbour the common deletion.

In the IBM group, all but one patient (89%) were found to harbour the common deletion.

Individual results of the patients are shown in table 2 column 3.

5.1.3 Real-time PCR: common deletion

In the control group the mean degree of common deletion was 0.03% (Range: 0-0.2%)

In the dermatomyositis group the mean degree of common deletion was 0.23% (Ramge: 0-2.48%)

In the polymyositis group the mean degree of common deletion was 0.14% (Ramge: 0-0.82%)

In the IBM group the mean degree of common deletion was 0.5% (Range: 0.03-1.45%)

Individual results of the patients are shown in table 2 column 3.

Table 2: Histological, biochemical and molecular findings in subjects and patients included in the study: (C1-C10 = controls, D1-D14 = Dermatomyositis patients, P1-P12 = polymyositis patients and I1-I9 = IBM patients)

Patients	Presence of multiple deletions in Long-Range -PCR	Presence of common deletion in CD PCR	Level of common deletion Real-time PCR (%)	COX/ CS activity* (%)	CNF** (%)	RRF** (%)
C1	normal	negative	0	73.49	0.3	1.8
C2	normal	negative	0	71.33	0.7	0
C3	weak	strong	0.05	62.24	0.1	0
C4	normal	negative	0	58.94	0.6	1.2
C5	weak	weak	0.04	58.12	0.3	2.1
C6	normal	negative	0	65.74	0.2	1.1
C7	normal	negative	0	53.99	0.5	3
C8	normal	negative	0	47.72	0.5	0
C9	normal	negative	0.04	114.46	0.9	0
C10	normal	negative	0.2	89.15	0.5	0.5
Total	*2/10*	*2/10*	*Mean: 0.03*	*Mean: 69.5*	*Mean: 0.46*	*Mean: 0.97*
D1	normal	negative	0	47.93	2.1	0
D2	strong	negative	0.01	47.03	2.7	3.4
D3	weak	strong	0.03	52.1	1.5	0
D4	normal	negative	0	98	5.2	0.2
D5	normal	negative	0	43.85	0.6	30.2
D6	weak	negative	0.29	45.91	1.3	3.3
D7	normal	strong	0.04	58.82	85.4	42.5
D8	weak	negative	0.06	77.71	1.6	1.6
D9	normal	strong	2.48	58.9	3.2	0.4
D10	strong	strong	0.14	19.88	2.2	25

D11	strong	negative	0.02	62.5	0.4	0.2
D12	normal	negative	0	64.29	1.2	0
D13	normal	negative	0.12	38.48	7.2	0.3
D14	weak	weak	0.01	74.47	0.9	0
Total	7/13	5/13	Mean: 0.23	Mean: 56.4	Mean: 17.5	Mean: 7.6
P1	normal	negative	0.03	44.14	0	1.4
P2	weak	strong	0.06	43.32	0.4	0.3
P3	normal	negative	0.12	63.03	0.1	2.5
P4	normal	negative	0.01	144.26	2	0.1
P5	weak	normal	0.04	68.99	0.5	0.8
P6	normal	negative	0	?	0.9	0.5
P7	normal	negative	0	36.4	0	0
P8	normal	negative	0.15	67.01	31.7	8.2
P9	normal	strong	0.12	105.2	17	9.3
P10	weak	strong	0.08	61.65	22.4	0.6
P11	strong	strong	0.82	56.25	12.5	1.6
P12	weak	weak	0.35	62.52	17.3	2.5
Total	5/12	5/12	Mean: 0.14	Mean: 68.3	Mean: 8.1	Mean: 2.2
I1	weak	strong	0.7	44.74	10.4	0.7
I2	weak	negative	0.03	73.64	2.5	10.1
I3	strong	strong	1.03	59.74	19.4	1.7
I4	weak	strong	0.14	64.82	3.4	0
I5	strong	strong	0.14	66.67	10.2	1
I6	weak	strong	1.45	119.95	8	0
I7	strong	strong	0.73	43.16	17	1.2
I8	strong	strong	0.2	82.36	13.4	2
I9	strong	strong	0.04	75.76	1.4	0.2
Total	9/9	8/9	Mean: 0.5	Mean: 70	Mean: 9.5	Mean: 1.9

CNF: COX deficient fibres, RRF: Ragged-red fibres, CD: Common deletion, CS: Citrate synthase, M: Male, F: Female, strong/weak: intensity of DNA bands in agarose gel, normal: no multiple deletions, negative: no common deletion

*: Ratio of COX (units/ gram dry weight) to citrate synthase (units/gram dry weight) in percentage.

**: CNF and RRF referred from the doctoral thesis of Dr. P. Tacik (Tacik, 2011).

5.1.4 Multiple-cell real-time PCR: common deletion

Multiple-cell real-time PCR analysis was done in randomly selected cases in control group (n=1) and myositis patients (DM=2, PM=2, IBM=3). The degrees of CD in individual normal- and COX negative fibres are listed in table 3.

Table 3: Results of multiple-cell real-time PCR of common deletion

Patient	CD deletion in COX negative fibres (%)	CD deletion in COX positive fibres (%)
C11	84	11
D9	95	33
D13	84	26
P2	83	7
P11	95	32
I6	98	37
I7	93	30
I9	94	26

CD: Common deletion, C: Control, D: Dermatomyositis, P: Polymyositis, I: inclusion body myositis

5.1.5 Level of common deletion in CPEO patients:

In order to optimise the real-time PCR analysis, CPEO patients with known levels of heteroplasmy of the common deletion in southern-blot analysis were used as controls for real-time PCR analysis. The levels of common deletion in both the methods are listed in table 4.

Table 4: Comparison of levels of deletion of the common deletion of CPEO patients in Southern-blot and real-time PCR analysis.

Patient Nr.	CD deletion in Southern-blot (%)	CD deletion in Real-Time (%)
1	28	18
2	30	26
3	32	29
4	48	30
5	60	59
6	65	62
7	40	36
8	50	47
9	50	44

CD: Common deletion

5.2 Biochemical results

Cytochrome c oxidase (COX) and citrate synthase (CS) activities were measured in the muscle homogenate of myositis patients and controls. The ratio of COX (units/gram dry weight) to CS (units/gram dry weight) was calculated and interpreted as percentage residual activity. In control group, the range of COX/CS activity was 47.72-114.46%. In dermatomyositis, the range of COX/CS activity was 18.88-98%. In polymyositis the range of COX/CS activity was 36.4-144.26%. In inclusion body myositis, the range of COX/CS activity was 43.16-119.95%. Individual results of of COX/CS activity are listed in table 2, column 5.

5.3 Comparison of different mitochondrial abnormalities

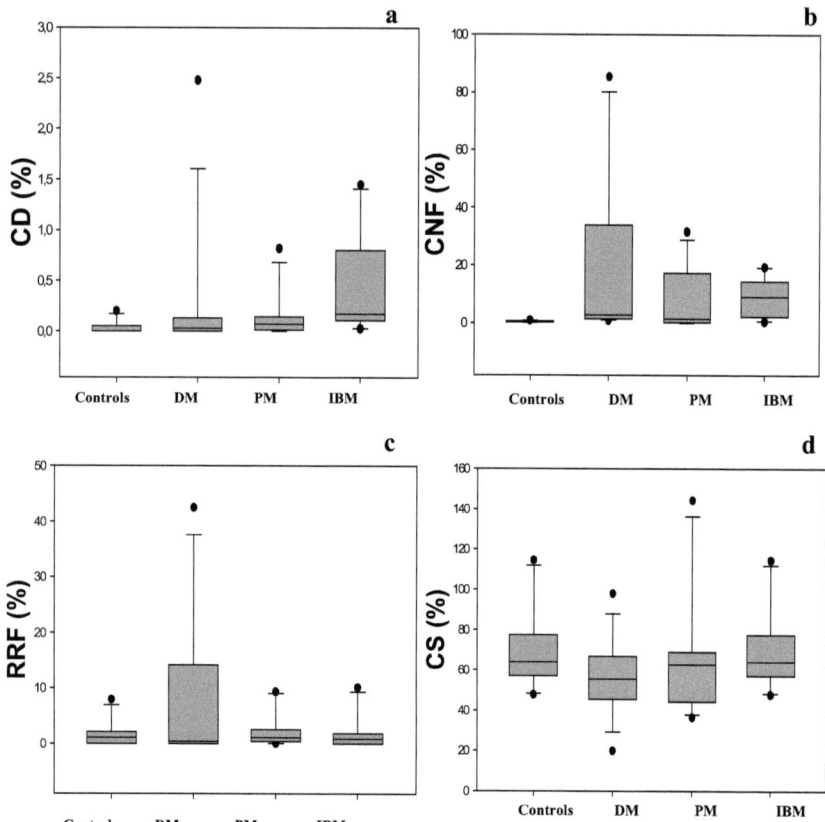

Figure 15: Box diagrams showing comparison of different mitochondrial abnormalities, viz., (a) levels of common deletion, (b) degree of COX negative fibres, (c) degree of ragged-red fibres, and (d) citrate synthase activity in control group and myositis patients. The upper and lower limits represent the range. The lower part of box represents 25th percentile and the upper part represents 75th percentile. The horizontal line bisecting the box represents the median. Percentage CS activity is the ratio of COX (units/gram dry weight) to Citrate synthase (units/gram dry weight).

6. Statistical analysis:

6.1 Comparison of levels of common deletion in CPEO patients in Southern-blot and real-time PCR

Correlation analysis between levels of CD in Southern-blot and real-time PCR analysis was done in CPEO patients. The statistical analysis using SPSS software shows a significant correlation in level of 0.01 (with Pearson's correlation coefficient: 0.94) (Appendix: Table A)

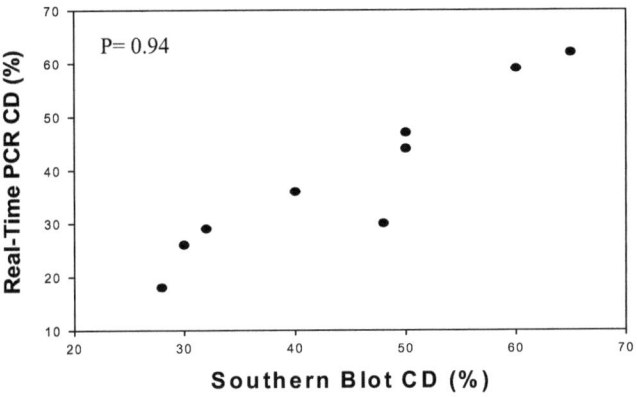

Figure 16: Correlation analysis of levels of common deletion in southern blot and real-time PCR analysis in CPEO patients.

6.2 2x2 contingency tables comparing molecular genetic abnormalities

Molecular genetic abnormalities (multiple deletions and common deletion) in patients with different forms of myositis were compared with abnormalities in normal controls by using 2x2 contingency tables. The P value was calculated with Fischer's exact test.

Table 5: 2x2 contingency table comparing molecular genetic abnormalities in controls and myositis patients

	Multiple deletions	Normal	Total	Common deletion	Normal	Total
Controls	2	8	10	2	8	10
Dermatomyositis	7	7	14	5	9	14
Total	9	15	24	7	17	24

Fisher's exact test: The two tailed P value for multiple deletions equals 0.1930 and for common deletion equals 0.3864

	Multiple deletions	Normal	Total	Common deletion	Normal	Total
Controls	2	8	10	2	8	10
Polymyositis	5	7	12	5	7	12
Total	7	15	22	7	15	22

Fisher's exact test: The two tailed P values for multiple deletions and common deletion equals 0.3707

	Multiple deletions	Normal	Total	Common deletion	Normal	Total
Controls	2	8	10	2	8	10
Inclusion body myositis	9	0	9	8	1	9
Total	11	8	19	10	9	19

Fisher's exact test: The two tailed P value for multiple deletions equals 0.0002 and for common deletion equals 0.0019

6.3 Comparison of degree of heteroplasmy of the common deletion

Levels of heteroplasmy obtained by real-time PCR analysis in muscle homogenates of patients with different forms of myositis were compared with levels of heteroplasmy in control group using Mann-Whitney rank sum test. The detailed result is shown in table 8.

Table 6: Mann-Whitney rank sum test comparing levels of heteroplasmy in patients with different forms of myositis with controls.

Groups	N	Missing	Median	25%	75%
Dermatomyositis	14	0	0.0300	0.000	0.125
Control	10	0	0.000	0.000	0.0475

T = 121.000 n (small) = 11 n (big) = 13
P = 0.353

Groups	N	Missing	Median	25%	75%
Polymyositis	12	0	0.0700	0.0200	0.135
Control	10	0	0.000	0.000	0.0475

T = 102.000 n (small) = 11 n (big) = 12
P = 0.069

Groups	N	Missing	Median	25%	75%
Inclusion body	9	0	0.170	0.130	0.730
Control	10	0	0.000	0.000	0.0475

T = 152.500 n (small) = 10 n (big) = 11
P = 0.003

6.4 Scatter plots:

Scatter plots comparing levels of common deletion in muscle homogenates in individual groups with age and histological and biochemical mitochondrial abnormalities were drawn, using Sigmaplot software.

6.4.1 Control Group:

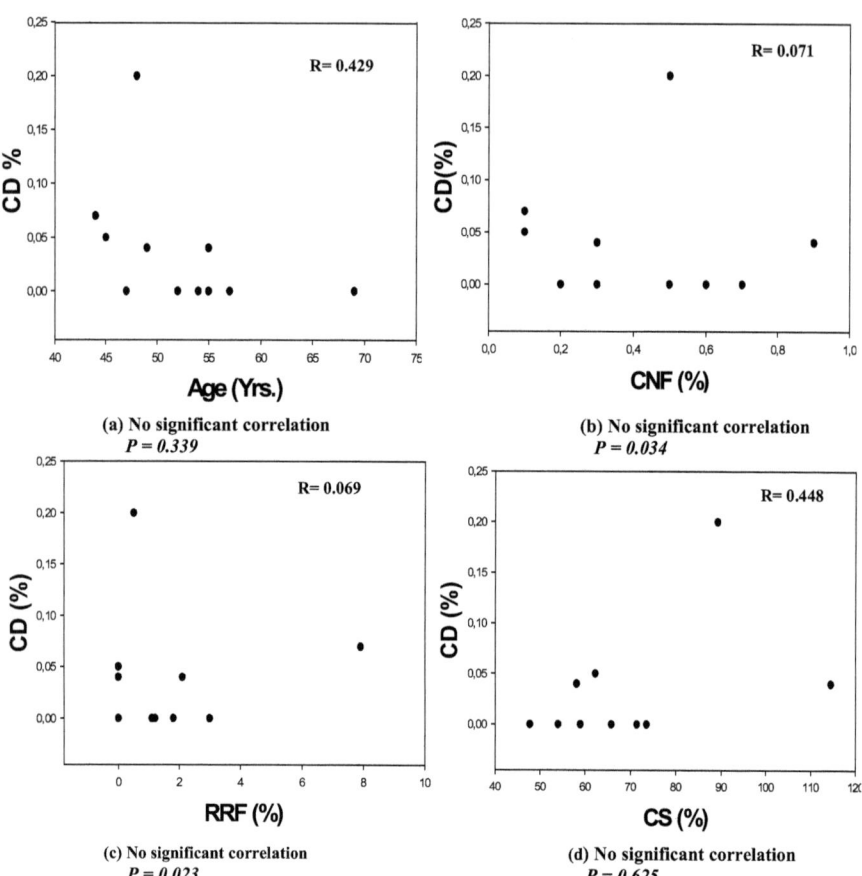

Figure 17: *Scatter plots comparing association of degree of common deletion with (a) age, (b) degree of COX negative fibres, (c) degree of ragged-red fibres, and (d) degree of citrate synthase activity in control group. CD: Common deletion, CNF: COX negative fibres, RRF: Ragged-red fibres, CS: Citrate synthase, R: Regression coefficient, P: Probability coefficient Percentage CS activity is the ratio of COX (units/gram dry weight) to Citrate synthase (units/gram dry weight).*

6.4.2 Dermatomyositis:

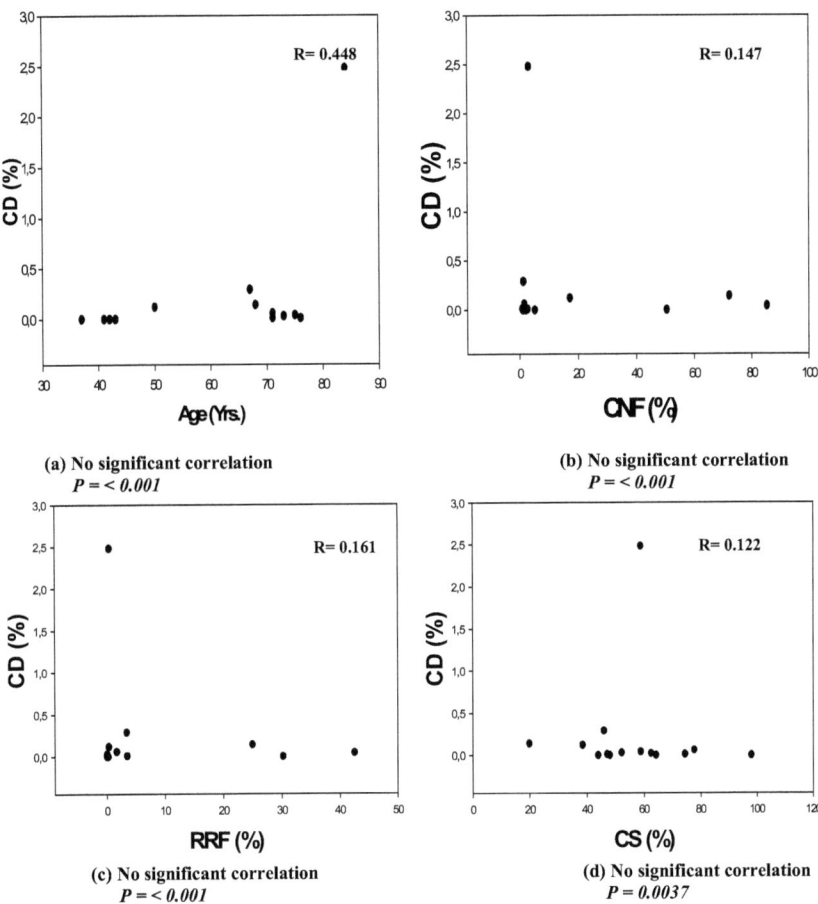

Figure 18: Scatter plots comparing association of degree of common deletion with (a) age, (b) degree of COX negative fibres, (c) degree of ragged-red fibres, and (d) degree of citrate synthase activity in dermatomyositis. CD: Common deletion, CNF: COX negative fibres, RRF: Ragged-red fibres, CS: Citrate synthase, R: Regression coefficient, P: Probability coefficient. Percentage CS activity is the ratio of COX (units/gram dry weight) to Citrate synthase (units/gram dry weight).

6.4.3 Polymyositis:

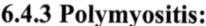

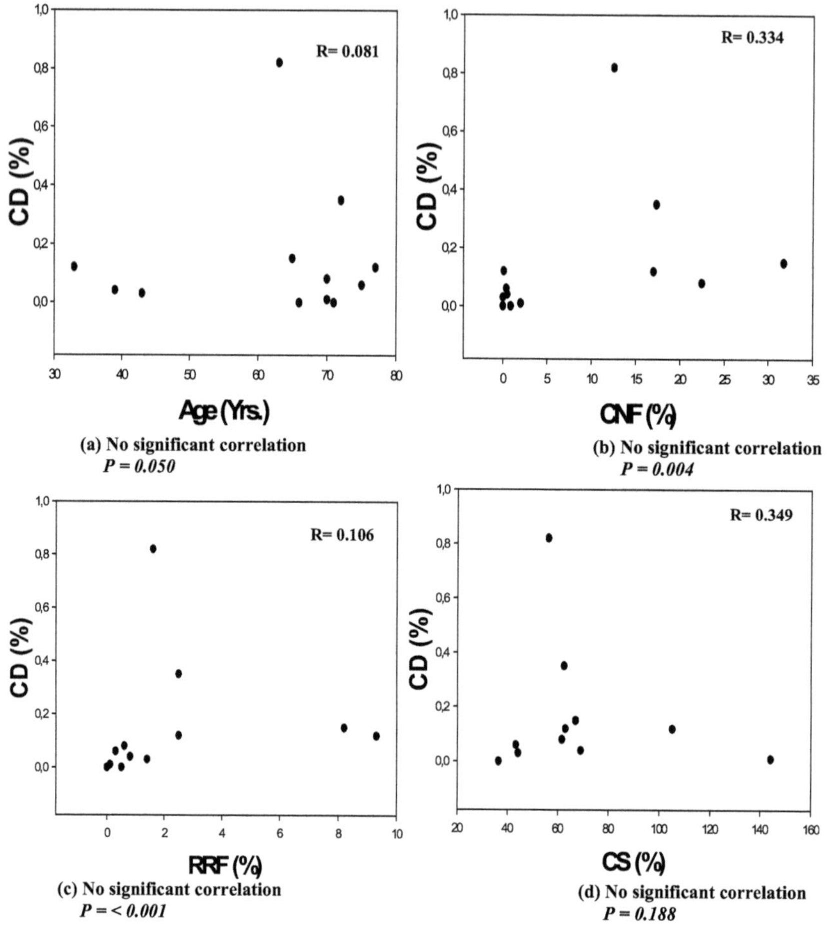

(a) No significant correlation
P = 0.050

(b) No significant correlation
P = 0.004

(c) No significant correlation
P = < 0.001

(d) No significant correlation
P = 0.188

Figure 19: *Scatter plots comparing association of degree of common deletion with (a) age, (b) degree of COX negative fibres, (c) degree of ragged-red fibres, and (d) degree of citrate synthase activity in polymyositis. CD: Common deletion, CNF: COX negative fibres, RRF: Ragged-red fibres, CS: Citrate synthase, R: Regression coefficient, P: Probability coefficient. Percentage CS activity is the ratio of COX (units/gram dry weight) to Citrate synthase (units/gram dry weight).*

6.4.4 Inclusion body myositis:

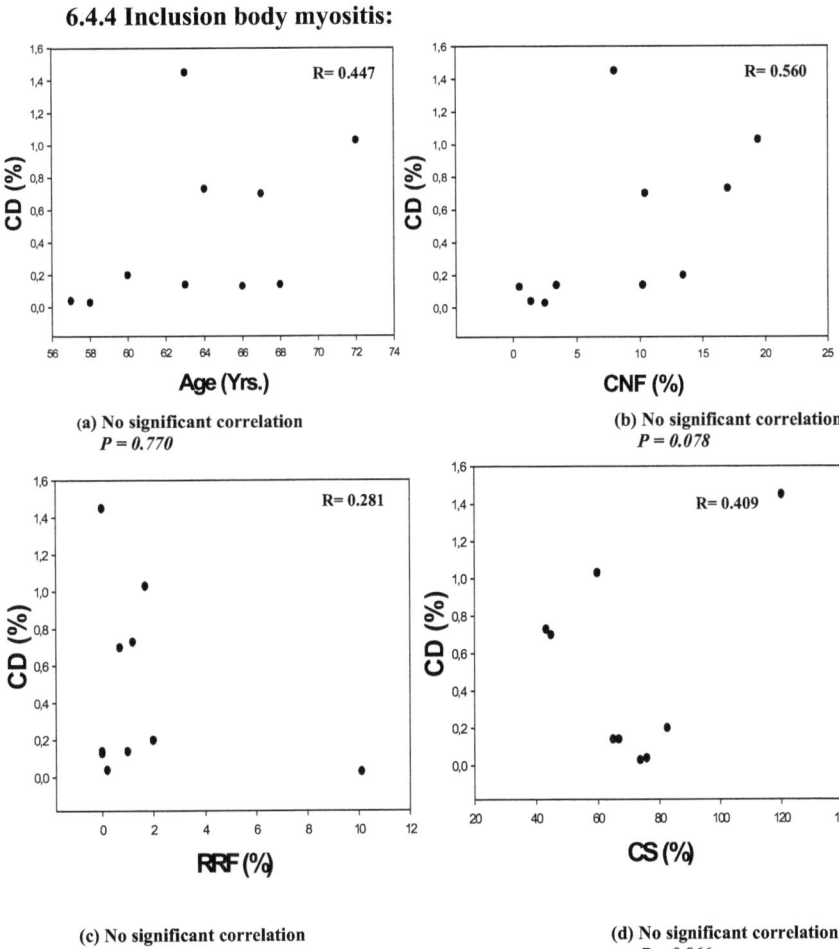

(a) No significant correlation
P = 0.770

(b) No significant correlation
P = 0.078

(c) No significant correlation
P = 0.067

(d) No significant correlation
P = 0.966

Figure 20: Scatter plots comparing association of degree of common deletion with (a) age, (b) degree of COX negative fibres, (c) degree of ragged-red fibres, and (d) degree of citrate synthase activity in inclusion body myositis. CD: Common deletion, CNF: COX negative fibres, RRF: Ragged-red fibres, CS: Citrate synthase, R: Regression coefficient, P: Probability coefficient. Percentage CS activity is the ratio of COX (units/gram dry weight) to Citrate synthase (units/gram dry weight).

6.5 Correlation analysis

Correlation analysis comparing different parameters (age, levels of common deletion, levels of COX negative fibres and levels of ragged-red fibres) was done within different groups (viz. control, DM, PM, and IBM), using SPSS software.

Apart from significant correlations at the levels 0.01 and 0.05 (Pearson's correlation coefficients: 0.959 and 0.667, respectively) between the levels of COX negative fibres and ragged-red fibres in DM and PM groups, respectively, no significant correlation was seen between different parameters within the individual groups. Detailed statistical report is tabulated in Appendix: Table B

6.6 Statistical comparison of molecular and histological changes

One way ANOVA test was performed to compare age and molecular and histological mitochondrial changes between- and within different groups, using SPSS software. No significant correlation was seen. Detailed statistical ANOVA result is tabulated in Appendix, table C.

7. Discussion

The current study aimed to identify a possible correlation between molecular genetic, biochemical and histological mtDNA abnormalities in different types of myositis with an emphasis on qualitative and quantitative aspects of mtDNA deletions. Clinically and histologically well characterised myositis patients (DM=14, PM=12, IBM=9) were included in the study with healthy individuals as normal controls (N=10).

The degree of mtDNA deletions in myositis patients being very low, deletions were not detected with Southern-blot analysis Previous studies also show that deletions were not seen with Southern-blot in IBM but all the patients had significant number of COX deficient fibres [Oldfors et al., 1993; Oldfors et al., 2006]. The specially designed, sensitive real-time PCR, however, did pick the common deletion (CD). As expected, the degree of this common deletion was very small (less than 1% in most of the cases) in muscle homogenate. Since the range of degrees of deletion was very small, it was obvious that a slight experimental error would change the outcome by a bigger dimension. In order to get maximum efficiency, the real-time PCR method was optimised by using CPEO patients (N=9) with comparatively higher degrees of the common deletion which was efficiently picked up also by the Southern-blot analysis. The corresponding degrees of deletion in CPEO patients obtained by both the methods; the real-time PCR method and the Southern-blot method, were comparable with a high statistical significance, indicating that the real-time PCR method was, in fact, reliable.

For qualitative analysis, specially designed 10 kb long-range PCR was performed to detect the multiple deletions. Additionally, a specific 'common deletion PCR' was designed to detect the common deletion. Weak multiple deletions and the common deletion DNA bands were seen in two of the control cases. In both of these cases, common deletion was also detected in small degrees by the quantitative real-time PCR. In addition, the real-time PCR did also detect the common deletion in three of the other control cases but the long-range PCR and the specific common deletion PCR were unable to detect the multiple deletions and the common deletion. Mitochondrial abnormalities could also be seen even in elderly healthy cases [Linnane et al., 1990; Katayama et al., 1991] but these three cases were not the oldest in the group. However, the oldest case in the control group (aged 69 years) had no multiple deletions and the common deletion in mitochondrial DNA and the real-time PCR also did not pick any common deletion. There were also a few cases in the myositis groups where the real-time PCR shows degrees of heteroplasmy of the common deletion but the long-range PCR and/or the specific common deletion PCR do not show the multiple deletions and/or the common deletion. This indicates that the long-range PCR and the specific common PCR are not that specific as is the quantitative real-time PCR. However, the long-range PCR and the specific common deletion PCR are efficient methods for qualitative analysis as these methods require less effort and time. Some general modifications in a way that smaller levels of deletions could be detected, would definitely make these qualitative methods more reliable and efficient. But, in any case, real-time PCR will remain the gold standard for quantitative DNA analysis.

MtDNA deletions are frequently reported in IBM [Oldfors et al., 1995; Moslemi et al., 1997; Amato and Shebert, 1998; Oldfors et al. 2006]. Similar to previous findings, multiple deletions were identified in all the IBM patients and the specific common deletion PCR detected the common deletion in all but one patient. The mean degree of common deletion in IBM patients was 0.5%, which was the highest among controls and other myositis patients. The range of the degree of common deletion was 0.03 to 1.45%. The result strengthens the fact that mtDNA deletions are quite frequent in IBM.

In polymyositis group, multiple deletions were identified in 4 patients who also harboured the common deletion. Apart from these four patients, two other patients also harboured only multiple deletions and the common deletion each. The mean degree of the common deletion in this group was 0.14% (range: 0-0.82%). There are not much data regarding mtDNA abnormalities in polymyositis but one previous study has identified deletions in two polymyositis cases [Molnar and Schröder, 1998]. Current findings show that deletions are also identified in patients with polymyositis but are not that frequent like in inclusion body myositis.

Multiple deletions and the common deletion were also detected in dermatomyositis patients. Three of the dermatomyositis patients harboured both the multiple deletions and the common deletion. Additionally, four additional patients had only multiple deletions and two other patients had only common deletion. The mean degree of common deletion in this groups was intermediate of the other two, polymyositis and inclusion body myositis groups, at 0.23% (range:0-2.48%). There are no data of mtDNA abnormalities in dermatomyositis in the literature. The current study shows that the mtDNA deletions are also fairly present in dermatomyositis. In fact, the frequency of mtDNA deletions in dermatomyositis is marginally higher than that in polymyositis.

The association of multiple deletions and common deletion with respect to the control groups and the groups with different forms myositis was analysed by calculating the two-tailed P value by Fischer's exact test using the 2x2 contingency table. The P values for multiple deletions in case of dermatomyositis and the polymyositis groups were 0.1930 and 0.3707 respectively. This shows that the association between the frequency of multiple deletions in dermatomyositis and polymyositis and that in control groups had no statistical significance. On the other hand, the P value for multiple deletions in inclusion body myositis against the control group was 0.0002, suggesting a very strong statistical significance.

Similarly, The P values for the common deletion in case of dermatomyositis and the polymyositis groups were 0.3864 and 0.3707 respectively. This shows that the association between the frequency of the common deletion in dermatomyositis and polymyositis and that in control groups had no statistical significance. However, the P value for the common deletion in IBM against the control group was 0.0019, suggesting a very strong statistical significance. This was similar as in case of multiple deletions in IBM.

Hence, the Fischer's exact test shows that the multiple deletions and the common deletion are more frequent in patients with IBM than in dermatomyositis and polymyositis and are statistically significant than that in normal healthy controls. This statistical finding strengthens the argument that the role of mtDNA deletions is more important in inclusion body myositis.

In order to correlate the degree of the common deletion obtained by real-time PCR, Mann-Whitney rank sum test was performed. The test showed that the difference in the median values between the control group and the dermatomyositis group was not great enough to exclude the possibility that the difference was due to random sampling variability, hence there was no statistically significant difference (P=0.353). Similarly, the difference in the median values in the control group and the polymyositis group was also not great enough to exclude the possibility that the difference was due to sampling variability suggesting that there was no statistically significant difference (P=0.069). Unlike in dermatomyositis group and the polymyositis group, the difference in the median values between the control group and the IBM group was greater than would have been expected by chance which suggested a statistically significant difference (P=0.003). Hence, the Mann-Whitney rank sum test shows that the degree of heteroplasmy of the common deletion plays a significant role in case of patients with IBM than in dermatomyositis and polymyositis. This statistical finding is totally in line with that of the Fischer's exact test which is in favour of the argument that the role of mtDNA deletions in myositis is more important in severity of IBM.

The degree of common deletion in the muscle homogenate of the myositis patients was very low (less than 1% in most of the cases). In order to analyse the presence of the common deletion in individual fibres, multiple-cell real-time analysis of the individual COX deficient and COX positive (normal) fibres was performed in at least two patients from each of the groups (DM, PM and IBM) and one patient from the control group. As expected, the degree of heteroplasmy of the common deletion was remarkably higher in the COX negative fibres than in the COX positive fibres. From the findings, the threshold for degree of presence of common deletion in a fibre to become COX deficient was roughly 80%. Previous studies have shown that the proportion of COX-negative fibres in a muscle section correspond broadly to the severity of a mitochondrial myopathy [Elson et al., 2002]. However, muscle fibres are large multi-nucleated cells that may be many centimetres in length, and it is well recognised that COX activity may vary along the length of muscle fibre [Elson et al., 2002] but the defined regions of COX deficiency have not been documented in muscles of myositis patients.

The exact correlation between the mtDNA deletions and the residual COX activity in myositis is not known. In order to compare the degrees of common deletion and the residual enzyme activity, the cytochrome c oxidase and the citrate synthase activities were measured in the muscle homogenate of all the controls and patients. The ratio of cytochrome c oxidase activity to the activity of citrate synthase was compared with the degrees of common deletion in each group. Statistical analysis, however, did not show any significant correlation in any of the groups of myositis and controls. This result shows that the deficiency of cytochrome c oxidase in myositis is not necessarily triggered by mtDNA deletions. The exact mechanism of enzyme deficiency in myositis is still unknown.

To compare the molecular genetic data of myositis patients, the histological results of the same patients was referred from the doctoral thesis of Pawel Tacik. Partial correlation analysis was also done by assuming age as an invariable factor and the degree of heteroplasmy of the common deletion, percentage of the COX negative fibres, and percentage of the ragged-red fibres by using SPSS software (version 16.0). Except for a significant correlation between percentage of COX negative fibres and the ragged-red fibres in dermatomyositis group (P = 0.958), no significant correlation was perceived in other groups. Previous study addressing IBM shows that there is no clear correlation between the degree of COX deficient fibres and muscle weakness or disease duration [Oldfors et al., 1993]. Our finding also shows that different forms of mitochondrial abnormalities are not significantly correlated with each other and hence one entity does not trigger the other. For example, it will not necessarily be the case that the patient having a considerable percentage of the COX negative fibres or the ragged-red fibres will also have a higher level of heteroplasmy of the common deletion and vice-versa.

However, in present study, a sub-group of polymyositis was identified with rather unsually high number of COX deficient fibres. In this sub-group, the mean frequency of COX deficient fibres was 20.18% in contrast to a total mean frequency of 8.1% and the partial mean frequency excluding this sub group, 0.06%. Only one patient in this COX deficient sub-group of polymyositis did not harbour both multiple deletions and the common deletion. Otherwise all the patients except one harboured, either, multiple deletions and/or the common deletion or the both. This was an interesting finding which shows that the deletions of mtDNA should be, in some capacity, responsible for COX deficiency in this sub-group of polymyositis.

The current study was unable to establish a concrete correlation between the mtDNA deletions and biochemical and histological mitochondrial abnormalities. Similarly, the exact correlation between mtDNA deletions and the mitochondrial abnormalities in myositis patients is of yet unknown. However, a study that addressed age-related mitochondrial alterations identified 50 different deletions in 30 subjects of different age [Pesce et al., 2001]. The study shows that some of these deletions were present only in few cases, others were frequent and the common deletion being most frequent. Furthermore, the percentage of the common deletion was directly proportional with the corresponding value of COX-negative and ragged-red fibres in each subject [Pesce et al., 2001]. However, the comparison did not show a direct correlation between the percentage of the common deletion and frequencies of COX-negative and ragged-red fibres suggesting a different mechanism of pathogenesis in myositis than in ageing.

In general, it has been found that the mitochondrial abnormalities develop with age [Linnane et al., 1990; Katayama et al., 1991]. In order to have an idea how the factor 'age' is related with the degree of heteroplasmy of the common deletion, a correlation analysis was done in the control group. Interestingly, no correlation was seen. The possible explanation of this outcome might be 'not-so-old' age of the subjects.

One but all the subjects were younger than 57 years and in terms of ageing, sixth decade of life can not be convincingly considered as aged. In similar manner, no significant correlation between age and the degree of heteroplasmy of the common deletion was seen in any of the myositis groups, either.

Pathogenesis of mtDNA deletions is not yet clearly understood but, deletions of tRNA genes in mitochondria containing only deleted mtDNAs are known to render the organelles incompetent for translation. Conversely, if a deletion does not contain the tRNA genes, the genetic defect may not manifest itself phenotypically. On the basis of these assumptions, Mita and co-workers have shown that mitochondria containing deleted genomes in PEO patients seemed to be competent for transcription but incompetent for translation and the COX deficiency in muscle sections from a patient with the common deletion was not segmental (i.e. normal in some regions of a fibre but deficient in others), but RNAs that were not encompassed by the deletion were transcribed but were not translated [Mita et al., 1990]. Based on these arguments, it is believed that large-scale deletions of mtDNA which remove structural genes but not any tRNA genes should result in a pathological phenotype characterized mainly by deficiency of just those specific respiratory chain enzyme activities corresponding to those subunit genes deleted in mtDNA. Moreover, mitochondria in such pathology would be competent for translation of the undeleted subunit gene transcripts and might not even proliferate and cause ragged-red fibres. The study shows that recombination via flanking direct repeats to be the main cause of large-scale deletions of mtDNA in patients with PEO [Mita et al., 1990].

Similar findings reported later in IBM patients indicate that there may be a common mechanism for the generation of mtDNA deletions in IBM and PEO patients [Moslemi et al., 1997]. Interestingly, nuclear factors have been implicated in the pathogenesis of both IBM [Griggs et al., 1995(b)] and PEO [Zeviani et al., 1990; Kaukonen et al., 1996]. Several factors involved in the replication, transcription, and maintenance of mtDNAs have been suggested to be involved in the pathogenesis of PEO [Zeviani et al., 1990; Larson and Clayton, 1995]. Such factors may thus also be involved in the pathogenesis of multiple mtDNA deletions in patients with different forms of myositis, although the consequences of any putative nuclear gene mutation may be indirect. The finding of clonal expansions of deleted mtDNA of the same types both in IBM [Kaukonen et al., 1996] and PEO [Mita et al., 1990] suggests that the deletions are not directly due to a single gene defect involved in the maintenance or replication of mtDNA. Factors that may damage mtDNA, such as oxygen radicals, are possibly of importance and have been suggested to cause mtDNA deletions in normal aging [Wei, 1992; Luft, 1994] and in PEO [Suomalainen et al., 1995]. Present study also shows multiple deletions in all IBM patients and most of the DM and PM patients which was quite contrasting to the normal controls. On the basis of finding of previous studies discussed afore, a speculation could be made that the same mechanisms promote the development of multiple mtDNA deletions in normal aging, IBM, PEO and other two forms of myositis (DM and PM), and the mechanisms are accentuated in PEO and IBM.

The inflammatory myopathies are auto-immune diseases and environmental factors are believed to trigger these diseases in genetically susceptible individuals. The specific causes or triggering events of the inflammatory myopathies are unknown but viruses have been implicated. A significant association between surface ultra violet exposure with the development of dermatomyositis was postulated [Okada et al., 2003; Birket et al., 2007].

The aetiology of myositis is unknown and the pathogenesis is only partly understood. An attack by T-lymphocytes on muscle fibres is considered to be of pathogenic importance [Arahata and Engel, 1988; Hohlfeld et al., 1991]. Additional factors, such as peripheral neuropathy, are also supposed to contribute disease purpose in inclusion body myositis [Eisen et al., 1983; Joy et al., 1990; Lindberg et al., 1990]. Ultra-structural mitochondrial changes [Carpenter et al., 1975] and ragged-red fibres [Carpenter and Karpati, 1984; Mikol, 1986] are seen to be common findings in muscle patients with IBM, in addition to the inflammatory infiltrates and rimmed vacuoles. Present findings with IBM were also in line with previous findings as all the IBM patients contained significant number of COX deficient fibres and the ragged-red fibres.

Since all the myositis patients contained COX deficient fibres in muscle and most of the patients also contained ragged-red fibres, these mitochondrial defects could be considered as one of the precursors of pathogenesis in myositis. Studies also report mitochondrial myopathies with ragged-red fibres being associated with large deletions of the mtDNA [Holt et al., 1988; Zeviani et al., 1988]. Large deletions of the mtDNA usually include several tRNA genes, which are necessary for mitochondrial protein synthesis. In many cases one or more of the three cytochrome c oxidase (COX) subunit genes encoded by the mtDNA are affected by the deletions [Moraes et al., 1989; Holt et al., 1989 (b)]. The deleted mtDNA and its transcripts are usually accumulated in muscle fibre segments, which show a reduced amount of normal mtDNA and deficient COX activity [Mita et al., 1989; Hammans et al., 1992(b); Oldfors et al., 1992]. A study conducted by Oldfors and co-workers did not find any clear correlation between the number of COX deficient fibres and muscle weakness or disease duration [Oldfors et al., 1993]. However, one case with severe inflammatory reaction showed the highest proportion of COX deficient fibres, and inflammatory infiltrates were frequently observed around or close to COX deficient fibres [Oldfors et al., 1993]. Similar to this finding, the results also show no clear correlation between the frequency of COX deficient fibres and other mitochondrial abnormalities.

As discussed, the pathogenesis of mtDNA deletions is not obvious due to heteroplasmy. The results of the multiple-cell PCR analysis that are discussed above, point out the drawbacks of the procedure we implemented in the beginning which gives more a virtual result than the real one. The DNA taken for the analysis of the common deletion was extracted from the muscle homogenates, which means a homogenous mixture of all the muscle fibres (normal and the COX negative) in the piece of muscle. On the other hand COX negative and the ragged-red fibres were counted manually on a section of slide which might not necessarily incorporate the same portion that is used for DNA extraction. Hence, the ideal method is to analyse the heteroplasmy level in single individual fibres. Similar findings are already reported that show an increased level of mtDNA deletion and low levels of wild-type mtDNA [Moraes et al., 1995]. Similar to current findings, the common deletion was identified in all fibres but in higher amounts in fibres with COX deficiency. These findings strengthen the argument that mitochondrial protein synthesis is impaired when a particular percentage of deletions in mtDNA is reached. However, the current results suggest that high levels of deletions in mtDNA alone do not seem to cause a severe COX deficiency and/or residual COX deficiency. Therefore, it is possible that the defect in mitochondrial protein synthesis is caused predominantly by the reduction of wild-type mtDNA in affected cells.

The study shows that whatever the cause of the mtDNA deletions in patients with different forms of myositis, the deletions may be of pathogenic significance and cause respiratory chain disfunction in segments of muscle fibres in muscle disorder.

8. Conclusions

Mitochondrial DNA deletions are seen in patients with different forms of myositis, being most prominent in IBM. Real-time PCR analysis is the ideal method to quantify very less levels of deletion with higher sensitivity. Apart from myositis patients, multiple deletions are also seen in some normal controls in Long-range PCR. The common deletion (CD) is also documented in some of the controls in Real-time PCR analysis but but the level of heteroplasmy is very less. Association between the frequency of the CD and multiple deletions in IBM with that in control group shows statistical significance. However no such significance was seen in case of DM and PM. No significant correlation was seen between reduced residual COX activity and the degree of CD in myositis patients and normal cases. Similarly, different forms of mitochondrial abnormalities (histological, biochemical, and genetic) are not significantly correlated with each other. However, all the myositis patients contained COX deficient fibres and most of the patients also had ragged-red fibres. Hence these mitochondrial defects could be considered as one of the precursors of pathogenesis in myositis.

Multiple-cell real-time PCR analysis detected CD in both normal and COX negative fibres. The levels of deletion were quite high than that in muscle homogenate. It was seen that the degree of presence of CD in a fibre to become COX negative is 80%. This suggests that mitochondrial protein synthesis is impaired when a particular percentage of deletions in mtDNA is reached. However, the high levels of deletions in mtDNA alone do not seem to cause a severe COX deficiency and/or residual COX deficiency.

9. References

Aaji C and Borst P. The gel electrophoresis of DNA. Biochim Biophys Acta. 1972;269:192-200

Alhatou MI, Sladky JT, Bagasra O, Glass JD. Mitochondrial abnormalities in dermatomyositis: characteristic pattern of neuropathology. J Mol Histol. 2004;35:615-619

Amato AA, Gronseth GS, Jackson CE, Wolfe GI, Katz JS, Bryan WW, Barohn RJ. Inclusion body myositis: clinical and pathological boundaries. Ann Neurol. 1996;40:581-586

Amato AA and Barohn RJ. Idiopathic inflammatory myopathies. Neurol Clin. 1997;15:615-648

Amato AA and Shebert RT. Inclusion body myositis in twins. Neurology. 1998;51:598-600

Anderson S, Bankier AT, Barrell BG, de Bruijn MHL, Coulson AR, Drouin J, Eperon IC, Nierlich DP, Roe BA, Sanger F, Schrier PH, Smith AJH, Staden R, Young IG. Sequence and organization of the human mitochondrial genome. Nature. 1981;290:457-465

Arahata K and Engel AG. Monoclonal antibody analysis of mononuclear cells in myopathies. I: Quantitative of subsets according to diagnosis and sites of accumulation and demonstration and counts of muscle fibres invaded by T cells. Ann Neurol. 1984;16:193-208

Arahata K and Engel AG. Monoclonal antibody analysis of mononuclear cells in myopathies. IV: Cell-mediated cytotoxicity and muscle fiber necrosis. Ann Neurol. 1988;23:168-173

Argov Z and Yarom R. ``Rimmed vacuole myopathy`` sparing the quadriceps: a unique disorder in Iranian Jews. J Neurol Sci. 1984;64:33-43

Askanas V, Engel WK, Alvarez RB. Enhanced detection of amyloid deposits in muscle fibres of inclusion body myositis and brain of Alzheimer disease using fluorescence technique. Neurology. 1993;43:1265-1267

Ballinger SW, Schoffner JM, Hedaya EV, et al. Maternally transmitted diabetes and deafness associated with 10.4 kb mitochondrial DANN deletion. Nat Genet.1992;1:11-15

Banker BQ. Dermatomyositis of childhood: ultrastructural alterations of muscle and intramuscular blood vessels. J Neuropathol Exp Neurol. 1975;34:46-75

Barnes WM. PCR amplification of up to 35-kb DNA with high fidelity and high yield from lambda bacteriophage templates. Proc Natl Acad Sci U S A. 1994;91(6):2216-2220

Barritt JA, Brenner CA, Cohen J, Watt DW. Mitochondrial DNA rearrangements in human oocytes and embryos. Mol Hum Reprod. 1999;5:927-933

Bender A, Krishnan KJ, Morris CM, Taylor GA, Reeve AK, Perry RH, Jaros E, Hersheson JS, Betts J, Klopstock T, Taylor RW, Turnbull DM. High levels of mitochondrial DNA deletions in substantia nigra neurons in aging and Parkinson disease. Nat Genet. 2006;38:515-517

Bernes SM, Bacino C, Prezant TR, Pearson MA, Wood TS, Fournier P, Fischel-Ghodsian N. Identical mitochondrial DNA deletion in mother with progressive external opthalmoplegia and son with Pearson marrow-pancrese syndrome. J Pediatr. 1993;123:598-602

Birket MJ, Birch-Machin MA. Ultraviolet radiation exposure accelerates the accumulation of the aging-dependent T414G mitochondrial DNA mutation in human skin. Aging Cell. 2007;6:557-564

Blakely EL, He L, Taylor RW, Chinnery P, Lightowlers RN, Schaefer AM, Turnbull DM. Mitochondrial DNA deletion in 'identical' twin brothers. J Med Genet. 2004;41

Bohan A and Peters JB. Polymyositis and dermatomyositis. Part 1. N Engl J Med. 1975;292:344-347

Bowmaker M, Yang MY, Yasukawa T, Reyes A, Jacobs HT, Huberman JA, Holt IJ. Mammalian mitochondrial DNA replicates bidirectionally from an initiation zone. J Biol Chem. 2003;278:50961-50969

Brown GK. Bottlenecks and beyond: mitochondrial DNA segregation in health and disease. J Inherit Metab Dis. 1997;20:2-8

Bruguier A, Texier P, Clement MC. Dermatomyositis infantiles : a propos de vingthuit observations. Arch Fr Pediatr. 1984; 41:9-14

Bua E, Johnson J, Herbst A, Delong B, McKenzie D, Salamat S, Aiken JM. Mitochondrial DNA-deletion mutations accumulate intracellularly to detrimental levels in aged human skeletal muscle fibres. Am J Hum Genet. 2006;469-480

Campos Y, Arenas J, Cabello A, Gomez-Reini JJ. Respiratory chain enzyme defects in patients with idiopathic inflammatory myopathy. Ann Rheum Dis. 1995;54:491-493

Carpenter S, Karpati G, Eisen A. A morphologic study in polymyositis: clues to pathogenesis of different types. 1975. In: Bradley W (ed) Recent advances in mycology. Excerpta Medica, Amsterdam, pp 374-379

Carpenter S and Karpati G. (eds.). Pathology of skeletal muscle(1984); New York: Churchill Livingstone

Chan CC, Liu VWS, Lau EYL, Yeung WSB, Ng EHY, Ho PC. Mitochondrial DNA content and 4977 bp deletion in unfertilized oocyte. Mol Hum Reprod. 2005;11:843-846

Chariot P, Ruet E, Authier FJ, Labes D, Poron F, Gherardi R. Cytochrome c oxidase deficiencies in the muscle of patients with inflammatory myopathies. Acta Neuropathol. 1996;91(5):530-536

Chen X, Prosser R, Simonetti S, Sadlock J, Jagiello G, Schon EA . Rearranged mitochondrial genomes are present in human oocytes. Am J Hum Genet 1995;57:239-247

Cheng S, Fockler C, Barnes WM, Higuchi R. Effective amplification of long targets from cloned inserts and human genomic DNA. Proc Natl Acad Sci U S A. 1994;91(12):5695-2699

Chinnery PF, DiMauro S, Shanske S, Schon EA, Zeviani M, Mariotti C, Carrara F, Lombes A, Laforet P, Ogier H, Jaksch M, Lochmüller H, Horvath R, Deschauer M, Thorburn DR, Bindoff LA, Poulton J, Taylor RW, Matthews JN, Turnbull DM. Risk of developing a mitochondrial DNA deletion disorder. Lancet. 2004;364:592-596

Chwalinska-Sadowska H and Madykowa H. Polymyositis-dermatomyositis: 25 year follow-up of 50 patients- disease course, treatment, prognostic factors. Mater Med Pol. 1990;22:213

Cook CD, Rosen FS, Banker BQ. Dermatomyositis and focal scleroderma. Pediatr Clin North Am. 1963;10:979-1016

Dalakas MC, Illa I, Pezeshkpour GH, Laukaitis JP, Cohen B, and Griffin JL. Mitochondrial myopathy caused by long-term zidovudine therapy. New Engl J Med. (1990);322:1098-1105

Dalakas MC. Polymyositis, dermatomyositis, and inclusion body myositis. N Engl J Med. 1991;325:1487-1498

Dalakas MC, Rakocevic G, Schmidt J, Salajegheh M, McElroy B, Harris-Love MO, Schrader JA, Levy EW, Dambrosia J, Kampen RL, Bruno DA, Kirk AD. Effect of Alemtuzumab (CAMPATH 1-H) in patients with inclusion-body myositis. Brain. 2009;132(Pt6):1536-1544

Darrow DH, Hoffman HT, Barnes GJ, Wiley CA. Management of dysphagia in inclusion body myositis. Arch Otolaryngol Head Neck Surg. 1992;118:313-317

DeVisser M, Emslie-Smith AM, Engel AG. Early ultrastructural alterations in dermatomyositis: capillary abnormalities precede other structural changes in muscle. J Neurol Sci. 1989;94:181-192

Doriguzzi C, Palmucci L, Pollo B, Mongini T, Maniscalco T, Chiado-Piat L, Schiffer D. Cytochrome c oxidase and coenzyme Q in neuromuscular diseases: a histochemical study. Acta Neuropathol. 1990;81:25-29

References

Dunbar DR, Moonie PA, Swingler RJ, Davidson D, Roberts R, Holt IJ. Maternally transmitted partial direct tandem duplication of mitochondrial DNA associated with diabetes mellitus. Hum Mol Genet. 1993;2:1619-1624

Eisen A, Berry K, Gibson G. Inclusion body myositis (IBM): myopathy or neuropathy? Neurology. 1983;33(9):1109-1114

Elson JL, Samuel DC, Johnson MA, Turnbull DM, Chinnery PF. The length od cytochrome c oxidase-negative segments in muscle fibres in patients with mtDNA myopathy. Neuromuscul Disord. 2002;12:858-864

Engel AG and Arahata K. Monoclonal antibody analysis of mononuclear cells in myopathies. II: Phenotypes of autoinvasive cells in polymyositis and inclusion body myositis. Ann Neurol. 1984;16:209-215

Engel AG, Hohlfeld B, Banker BQ. The polymyositis and dermatomyositis syndromes. In AG Engel, C Franzini-Armstrong (eds), Myology (2nd ed). New York: McGraw-Hill 1994;1335-1383

Griggs RC, Mendell JR, Miller RG. Inflammatory myopathies. In Evaluation and treatment of myopathies. Philadelphia: FA Davis, 1995(a);154-210

Griggs RC, Askanas V, DiMauro S, Engel A, Karpati G, Mendell JR, Rowland LP. Inclusion body myositis and myopathies. Ann Neurol. 1995 (b);38:705-713

Haber JE. Partners and pathways repairing a double-strand break. Trends Genet. 2000;16:259-264

Hammans SR, Sweeney MG, Wicks DAG, Morgan-Hughes JA, Harding AE. A molecular genetic study of focal histochemical defects in mitochondrial encephalomyopathies. Brain. 1992 (a);US:343-365

Hammans SR, Sweeny MG, Holt IJ, Cooper JM, Toscano A, Clark JB, Morgan-Hughes JA, Harding AE. Evidence of mitochondrial complementation between deleted and normal mitochondrial DNA in some patients with mitochondrial myopathy. J Neurol Sci. 1992 (b);107:87-92

Harding AE, Sweeney MG, Miller DH, Mumford CJ, Kellar-Wood H, Menard D, McDonald WI, Compston DAS. Occurence of a multiple sclerosis-like illness in women who have a Leber's hereditary optic neuropathy mitochondrial DNA mutation. Brain. 1992;115:979-989

Hayashi J, Ohta S, Kikuchi A, Takemitshu M, Goto Y-I, Nonaka I. Introduction of disease-related mitochondrial DNA deletions into HeLa cells lacking mitochondrial DNA results in mitochondrial dysfunction. Proc Natl Acad Sci USA. 1991;88:10614-10618

He L, Chinnery PF, Durham SE, Blakely EL, Wardell TM, Borthwick GM, Taylor RW, Turnbull DM. Detection and quantification of mitochondrial DNA deletions in individual cells by real-time PCR. Nucl Acid Res. 2002;30:e68

Helling RB, Goodman HM, Boyer HW. Analysis of endonuclease R-EcoRI fragments of DNA from lambdoid bacteriophages and other viruses by agarose-gel electrophoresis. J Virol. 1974;14(5):1235-1244

Hohlfeld R, Engel AG, Ii K, Harper MC. Polymyositis mediated by T-lymphocytes that express the gamma/delta receptor. N Engl J Med. 1991;324(13):877-881

Holt IJ, Harding AE, Morgan Hughes JA. Deletions of muscle mitochondrial DNA in patients with mitochondrial myopathies. Nature. 1988;331:717-719

Holt IJ, Harding AE, Cooper JM, Schapira AHV, Toscano A, Clark JB, Morgan-Hughes JA. Mitochondrial myopathies: clinical and biochemical features of 30 patients with major deletions of muscle mitochondrial DNA. Ann Neurol. 1989(a);26:699-708

Holt IJ, Harding AE, Morgan-Hughes JA. Deletions of muscle mitochondrial DNA in mitochondrial myopathies: sequence analysis and possible mechanisms. Nucleic Acids Res. 1989(b);17:4465-4469

Holt IJ, Dunbar DR, Jacobs HT. Behaviour of a population of partially duplicated mitochondrial DNA molecules in cell culture: segregation, maintenance and recombination dependent upon nuclear background. Hum Mol Genet 1997;6:1251-1260

Holt IJ, Lorimer HE and Jacobs HT. Coupled leading- and lagging-strand synthesis of mammalian mitochondrial DNA. Cell. 2000;100:515-524

Hudson G and Chinnery PF. Mitochondrial DNA polymerase-gamma and human disease. Hum Mol Genet. 2006;15:R244-252

Joffe MM, Love LA, Leff RL. Drug therapy of idiopathic inflammatory myopathies: predictors of response to prednisone, azathioprine, and methotrexate and a comparision of their efficacy. Am J Med. 1993;94:379-387

Joy JL, Oh SJ, Baysal AI. Electrophysiological spectrum of inclusion body myositis. Muscle Nerve. 1990;13:949-51

Katayama M, Tanaka M, Yamamoto H, Ohbayashi T, Nimura Y, Ozawa T. Deleted mitochondrial DNA in the skeletal muscle of aged individuals. Biochem Int. 1991;25:47-56

Kaukonen JA, Amati P, Suomalainen A, Rötig A, Piscaglia M-G, Salvi F, Weissenbach J, Fratta G, Comi G, Peltonen L, Zevianni M. An autosomal locus predisposing to multiple deletions of mtDNA on chromosome 3p. Am J Hum Genet. 1996;58:763-769

Krishnan KJ, Reeve AK, Samuels DC, Chinnery PF, Blackwood JK, Taylor RW, Wanrooij S, Spelbrink JN, Lightowlers RN, Turnbull DM.

What causes mitochondrial DNA deletions in human cells? Nat Genet. 2008;40:275-279

Kraytsberg Y, Kudryavtseva E, McKee AC, Geula C, Kowall NW, Khrapko K. Mitochondrial DNA deletions are abundant and cause functional impairment in aged human substantia nigra neurons. Nat Genet. 2006;38:518-520

Larson NG, Holmes E, Kristiansson B, Oldfors A, Tulinius M. Progressive increase of the mutated mitochondrial DNA fraction in Kearns-Sayre syndrome. Pediatr Res. 1990;28:131-136

Larsson NG and Clayton DA. Molecular genetic aspects of human mitochondrial disorders. Annu Rev Genet. 1995;29:151-178

Lertrit P, Kapsa RM, Jean-Francois MJ, Thyagarajan D, Noer AS, Marzuki S, Byrne E. Mitochondrial DNA polymorphism in disease: a possible contributor to respiratory dysfunction. Hum Mol Genet. 1994;3:1973-1981

Lindberg C, Oldfors A, Hedström A. Inclusion body myositis: peripheral nerve involvement. Combined morphological and electrophysiological studies in peripheral nerve. J Neurol Sci. 1990;99:327-338

Linnane AW, Baumer A, Maxwell RJ, Preston H, Zhang CF, Marzuki S. Mitochondrial gene mutation: the ageing process and degenerative diseases. Biochem Int. 1990;22:1067-1076

Lotz BP, Engel AG, Nishino H, Stevens JC, Litchy WJ. Inclusion body myositis. Observations in 40 patients. Brain;1989:112:727-747

Luft R. The development of mitochondrial medicine. Proc Natl Acad Sci USA. 1994;91:8731-8738

Manfredi G, Vu T, Bonilla E, Schon EA, DiMauro S, Arnaudo E, Zhang L, Rowland LP, Hirano M. Association of myopathy with large-scale mitochondrial DNA duplications and deletions: which is pathogenic? Ann Neurol. 1997;42:180-188

McFarland R, Chinnery PF, Blakely EL, Schaefer AM, Morris AAM, Foster SM, Tuppen HAL, Ramesh V, Dorman PJ, Turnbull DM, Taylor R. Homoplasmy, heteroplasmy, and mitochondrial dystonia. Neurology. 2007;69:911-916

Medsger TA Jr, Dawson WN, Masi AT. The epidemiology of polymyositis. Am J Med. 1970;48:715-723

Mikol J. Inclusion body myositis. In: Myology: basic and clinical. Edited by AG Engel and BQ Banker. 1986; New York: McGraw-Hill, pp 1423-1438

Mikol J and Engel AG. Inclusion body myositis. In AG Engel, C Franzini-Armstrong (eds), Myology (2nd ed). New York: McGraw-Hill, 1994;1384-1398

Miro O, Casademont J, Grau JM, Jarreta D, Urbano-Marquez A, Cardellach F. Histological and biochemical assessment of mitochondrial function in dermatomyositis. Br J Rheumatol. 1998;37:1047-1053

Mita S, Schmidt B, Schon EA, DiMauro S, Bonilla E. Deletion of ``deleted`` mitochondrial genomes in cytochrome-c oxidase-deficient muscle fibres of a patient with Kearns-Sayre syndrome. Proc Natl Acad Sci USA. 1989;86:9509-9513

Mita S, Rizzuto R, Moraes CT, Shanske S, Arnaudo E, Fabrizi GM, Koga Y, DiMauro S, Schon EA. Recombination via flanking direct repeats in a major cause of large-scale deletions of human mitochondrial DNA. Nucl Acid Res.1990;18:561-7

Molnar M and Schröder JM. Pleomorphic mitochondrial and different filamentous inclusions in inflammatory myopathies associated with mtDNA deletions. Acta Neuropathol. 1998;96:41-51

Moraes CT, DiMauro S, Zeviani M, Lombes A, Shanske S, Miranda AF, Nakase H, Bonilla E, Werneck LC, Servidei S. Mitochondrial DNA deletions in progressive external opthalmoplegia and Kearns-Sayre syndrome. N Engl J Med. 1989;320:1293-1299

Moraes CT, Sciacco M, Ricci E, Tengan CH, Hao H, Binilla E, Schon EA, DiMauro S. Phenotype-genotype correlations in skeletal muscle of patients with mtDNA deletions. Muscle Nerve. 1995;Suppl. 3:S150-153

Moslemi AR, Lindberg C, Oldfors A. Analysis of multiple mitochondrial DNA deletions in inclusion body myositis. Hum Mut. 1997;10:381-386

Mullis B and Faloona FA. Specific synthesis of DNA in vitro via a polymerase-catalysed chain reaction. Methods Enzymol. 1987;155:335-350

Nadege B, Patrick L, Rodrigue R. Mitochondria: from bioenergetics to the metabolic regulation of carcinogenesis. Front Biosci. (2009);14:4015-4034

Nguyen LH, Erzberger JP, Root J, Wilson DM. The human homolog of *Escherichia coli* Orn degrades small single-stranded RNA and DNA oligomers. J Biol Chem. 2000;275:25900-25906

Okada S, Weatherhead E, Targoff IN, Wesley R, Miller FW. Global surface ultraviolet radiation intensity may modulate the clinical and immunologic expression of autoimmune muscle disease. Arthritis Rheum. 2003;48:2285-2293

Oldfors A, Larsson N-G, Holme E, Tulinius M, Kadenbach D, Droste M. Mitochondrial DNA deletions and cytochrome c oxidase deficiency in muscle fibres. J Neurol Sci. 1992;110:169-177

Oldfors A, Larsson N-G, Lindberg C, Holme E. Mitochondrial DNA deletions in inclusion body myositis. Brain. 1993;116(Pt 2):325-336

Oldfors A, Moslemi AR, Fyhr IM, Holme E, Larsson N-G, Lindberg C. Mitochondrial DNA deletions in muscle fibers in inclusion body myositis. J Neuropathol Exp Neurol. 1995;54(4):581-7

Oldfors A, Moslemi AR, Jonasson L Ohlson M, Kollberg G, Lindberg C. Mitochondrial abnormalities in inclusion-body myositis. Neurology. 2006;66:S49-55

Pachman LM. Juvenile dermatomyositis. Pathophysiology and disease expression. Pediatr Clin North Am. 1995;42:1071-1098

Pesce V, Cormio A, Fracasso F, Vecchiet J, Felzani G, Lezza AMS, Cantatore P, Gadaleta MN. Age related mitochondrial genotypic and phenotypic alterations in human skeletal muscle. Free Radic Biol Med. 2001;30:1223-1233

Poulton J, Deadman ME, Gardiner RM. Duplications of mitochondrial DNA in mitochondrial myopathy. Lancet. 1989;1:236-240

Reeve AK, Krishnan KJ, Elson JL, Morris CM, Bender A, Lightowlers RN, Turnbull DM. Nature of mitochondrial DNA deletions in substantia nigra neurons. Am J Hum Genet. 2008;82:228-235

Rifai Z, Welle S, Kamp C, Thornton CA. Ragged red fibers in normal aging and inflammatory myopathy. Ann Neurol. 1995;37:24-29

Robberson DL and Clayton DA. Replication of mitochondrial DNA in mouse L cells and their thymidine kinase- derivatives: displacement replication on a covalently-closed circular template. Proc Natl Acad Sci USA. 1972;69:3810-3814

Rötig A, Bessis JL, Romero N, Cormier V, Saudubray J-M, Narcy P, Lenoir G, Rustin P, Munnich A. Maternally inherited duplication of the mitochondrial genome in a syndrome of proximal tubulopathy, diabetes mellitus, and cerebellar ataxia. Am J Hum Genet. 1992;50:364-370

Sabunciyan S, Kirches E, Krause G, Bogerts B, Mawrin C, Llenos IC, Weis S. Quantification of total mitochondrial DNA and mitochondrial common deletion in the frontal cortex of patients with schizophrenia and bipolar disorder. J Neural Transm. 2007;114:665-674

Sambrook J and Russel DW. Southern blotting: capillary transfer of DNA to membranes. Molecular Cloning, 3rd edition, by Joseph Sambrook and David W. Russell. Cold Spring Harbor Laboratory Press, Cold Spring Harbor, NY, USA, 2001

Samuels DC, Schon EA, Chinnery PF. Two direct repeats cause most human mtDNA deletions. Trends Genet. 2004;20:393-398

Schaefer AM, McFarland R, Blakely EL, He L, Whittaker RG, Taylor RW, Chinnery PF, Turnbull DM. Prevalence of mitochondrial DNA disease in adults. Ann Neurol. 2008;63:35-39

Servidei S. Mitochondrial encephalomyopathies: gene mutation. Neuromuscul Disord. 2003;13:277-282

Shoffner JM, Lott MT, Voljavec AS, Soueidan SA, Costigan DA, Wallace DC. Spontaneous Kearns-Sayre/chronic external opthalmoplegia plus syndrome associated with a mitochondrial DNA deletion: a slip-replication model and metabolic therapy. Proc Natl Acad Sci USA. 1989;86:7952-7956

Suelmann R and Fischer R. Mitochondrial movement and morphology depend on an intact actin cytoskeleton in Aspergillus nidulans. Cell Motil Cytoskeleton. 2000; 45:42-50

Suomalainen A, Kaukonen J, Amati P, et al. An autosomal locus predisposing to deletion of mitochondrial DNA. Nat Genet. 1995;9:146-51

Superti-Furga A, Schoenle E, Tuchschmid P, Caduff R, Sabato V, DeMattia D, Gitzelmann R, Steinmann B. Pearson bone marrow-pancreas syndrome with insulin-dependent diabetes, progressive renal tubulopathy, organic aciduria and elevated fetal haemoglobin caused by deletion and duplication of mitochondrial DNA. Eur J Pediatr. 1993;152:44-50

Tacik P. Myohistologische mitochondriale Veränderungen bei Patienten mit idiopathischen Myositiden. Halle Univ., Med. Fak., Diss. (2011)

Taylor RW, Barron MJ, Borthwick GM, Gospel A, Chinnery PF, Samuels DC, Taylor GA, Plusa SM, Needham SJ, Greaves LC, Kirkwood TBL,

Turnbull DM. Mitochondrial DNA mutations in human colonic crypt stem cells. J Clin Invest. 2003;112:1351-1360

Taylor RW and Turnbull DM. Mitochondrial DNA mutations in human disease. Nat Rev Genet. 2005;6:389-402

Tymms KE and Webb J. Dermatomyositis and other connective tissue diseases: a review of 105 cases. J Rheumatol. 1985;12:1140-1148

Wallace DC, Singh G, Lott MT, Hodge JA, Schurr TG, Lezza AMS, Elsas II LJ, Nikoskelainen EK. Mitochondrial DNA mutation associated with Leber's hereditary optic neuropathy. Science. 1988;242:1427-1430

Wang GJ, Nutter LM, Thayer SA. Insensitivity of cultured rat cortical neurons to mitochondrial DNA synthesis inhibitors: evidence for a slow turnover of mitochondrial DNA. Biochem Pharmacol. 1997;54:181-187

Wanrooji S, Luoma P, van Goethem G, van Broeckhoven C, Suomalainen A, Spelbrink JN. Twinkle and POLG defects enhance age-dependent accumulation of mutations in the control region of mtDNA. Nucleic Acid Res. 2004;32:3053-3064

Watkins SC and Cullen MJ. A qualitative and quantitative study of the ultrastructure of regenerating muscle fibres in Ducheme muscular dystrophy and polymyositis. J Neurol Sci. 1987;82:181-192

Wei YH. Mitochondrial DNA alterations as ageing-associated molecular events. Mutat Res. 1992;275:145-155

Yamamoto M, Koga Y, Ohtaki E, Nonaka I. Focal cytochrome c oxidase deficiency in various neuromuscular diseases. J Neurol Sci. 1989;91:207-213

Yang MY, Bowmaker M, Reyes A, Vergani L, Angeli P, Gringeri P, Jacobs HT, Holt IJ. Biased incorporation of ribonucleotides on the mitochondrial L-strand accounts for apparent strand-asymmetric DNA replication. Cell. 2002;111:495-505

Yasukawa T, Reyes A, Cluett TJ, Yang M-Y, Bowmaker M, Jacobs HT; Holt IJ. Replication of vertebrate mitochondrial DNA entails transient ribonucleotide incorporation throughout the lagging strand. EMBO J. 2006;25:5358-5371

Zeviani M, Moraes CT, DiMauro S, Nakase H, Bonilla E, Schon EA, Rowland LP. Deletions of mitochondrial DNA in Kearns-Sayre syndrome. Neurology. 1988;38:1339-1346

Zeviani M, Servidei S, Gellera C, Bertini E, DiMauro S, DiDonato S. An autosomal dominant disorder with multiple deletions of mitochondria starting at the D-loop region. Nature. 1989;339:309-311

Zeviani M, Bresolin N, Gellera C, Bordoni A, Pannacci M, Amati P, Moggio M, Servidei S, Scarlato G, DiDonato S. Nucleus-driven multiple large-scale deletions of the human mitochondrial genome: a new autosomal dominant disease. Am J Hum Genet. 1990;47:904-914

Appendix

A. Preparation of reagents:

Incubation medium:
10 mg DAB
9 ml 0.05 M sodium phosphate buffer at pH 7.4
750 mg Saccharose
2ml catalase 1:1000 in Bidest
20 mg cytochrome C

SDH solution:
100 µl sodium succinate
100 µl PMS
10 µl sodium azide
mixed to 800 µl NBT and vortexed

0.05 M phosphate buffer pH 7.4
$Na_2H_2PO_4$ (MW: 137.99)   6.9 g in 1000 ml Aquadest, pH adjusted to 7.4

0.1M phosphate buffer pH 7.0
$Na_2H_2PO_4$ (MW: 137.99)   1.38 g in 100 ml aquadest, pH adjusted to 7.0

130 mM sodium succinate (disodium salt). 6H2O (MW: 270.1)
350 mg in 10 ml 0.1 M sodium phosphate buffer, pH 7.0

1.875 mM Nitro blue tetrazolium (NBT) (MW: 817.6)

91.9 mg in 60 ml 0.1 M sodium phosphate buffer, pH 7.0

2 mM Phenazine methosulphate (PMS) (MW: 306.3) →

Sensitive to light!

6.13 mg in 10 ml 0.1 M sodium phosphate buffer. pH 7.0

100 mM sodium azide (MW: 65.01)

65 mg in 10 ml 0.1 M sodium phosphate buffer, pH 7.0

Assay Buffer (pH 7.0)	(with 1M HCl in 100ml)
10mM Tris-HCl	121.1 mg
(MW: 121.1 from Sigma (1Kg)	
120mM KCL	894.72 mg
(MW: 74.56 from Merck (1Kg)	

Enzyme diluting Buffer (pH 7.0)	(with 1M HCl in 25ml)
10 mM Tris-HCl	30.28 mg
250 mM Sucrose	2.139 g
(Sucrose Sigma Ultra 99.5% GC, MW: 342.3 from Sigma (250 g)	
1mM n-Dodecyl ß-D-Maltosid	12.77 mg
(MW: 510.63 from Sigma (1g)	

B. Statistical analysis (SPSS software)

Table A: Correlation analsis of levels of common deletion in southern-blot and real-time PCR analysis in CPEO patients

		Southern	Real-Time
Southern	Correlation (Pearson	1	0.940(**)
	Significance)		0.000
	N	9	9
Real-Time	Correlation (Pearson	0.940(**)	1
	Significance)	0.000	
	N	9	9

** The correlation is significant in level of 0.01.

Table B: Correlation analysis comparing different parameters (age, levels of common deletion, levels of COX negative fibres and levels of ragged-red fibres) within different groups (viz. control, DM, PM, and IBM).

Appendix

i. Control group:

Correlations

		Age	CD%	CNF%	RRF%
Age	Pearson Correlation	1	-0.429	0.102	-0.282
	Sig. (2-tailed)		0.188	0.766	0.400
	N	11	11	11	11
CD%	Pearson Correlation	-0.429	1	-0.072	0.070
	Sig. (2-tailed)	0.188		0.834	0.839
	N	11	11	11	11
CNF%	Pearson Correlation	0.102	-0.072	1	-0.488
	Sig. (2-tailed)	0.766	0.834		0.127
	N	11	11	11	11
RRF%	Pearson Correlation	-0.282	0.070	-0.488	1
	Sig. (2-tailed)	0.400	0.839	0.127	
	N	11	11	11	11

Descriptive Statistics

	Mean	Std. Deviation	N
Age	52.27	7.058	11
CD%	0.0364	0.06005	11
CNF%	0.4273	0.25334	11
RRF%	1.6000		11

ii. Dermatomyositis:

Correlations

		Age	CD%	CNF%	RRF%
Age	Pearson Correlation	1	0.448	0.074	0.087
	Sig. (2-tailed)		0.125	0.809	0.778
	N	13	13	13	13
CD%	Pearson Correlation	0.448	1	-0.147	-0.161
	Sig. (2-tailed)	0.125		0.631	0.599
	N	13	13	13	13
CNF%	Pearson Correlation	0.074	-0.147	1	0.959**
	Sig. (2-tailed)	0.809	0.631		0.000
	N	13	13	13	13
RRF%	Pearson Correlation	0.087	-0.161	0.959**	1
	Sig. (2-tailed)	0.778	0.599	0.000	
	N	13	13	13	13

**. Correlation is significant at the 0.01 level (2-tailed).

Descriptive Statistics

	Mean	Std. Deviation	N
Age	61.38	16.225	13
CD%	0.2446	0.67681	13
CNF%	18.8538	29.99841	13
RRF%	8.2231	14.40354	13

iii. Polymyositis

Correlations

		Age	CD%	CNF%	RRF%
Age	Pearson Correlation	1	0.081	0.399	0.165
	Sig. (2-tailed)		0.802	0.199	0.609
	N	12	12	12	12
CD%	Pearson Correlation	0.081	1	0.334	0.106
	Sig. (2-tailed)	0.802		0.289	0.742
	N	12	12	12	12
CNF%	Pearson Correlation	0.399	0.334	1	0.667*
	Sig. (2-tailed)	0.199	0.289		0.018
	N	12	12	12	12
RRF%	Pearson Correlation	0.165	0.106	0.667*	1
	Sig. (2-tailed)	0.609	0.742	0.018	
	N	12	12	12	12

*. Correlation is significant at the 0.05 level (2-tailed).

Descriptive Statistics

	Mean	Std. Deviation	N
Age	62.00	14.954	12
CD%	0.1483	0.23253	12
CNF%	8.7333	11.04193	12
RRF%	2.3167	3.12899	12

iv. Inclusion body myositis

Correlations

		Age	CD%	CNF%	RRF%
Age	Pearson Correlation	1	0.447	0.436	-0.407
	Sig. (2-tailed)		0.195	0.208	0.243
	N	10	10	10	10
CD%	Pearson Correlation	0.447	1	0.560	-0.281
	Sig. (2-tailed)	0.195		0.092	0.431
	N	10	10	10	10
CNF%	Pearson Correlation	0.436	0.560	1	-0.123
	Sig. (2-tailed)	0.208	0.092		0.734
	N	10	10	10	10
RRF%	Pearson Correlation	-0.407	-0.281	-0.123	1
	Sig. (2-tailed)	0.243	0.431	0.734	
	N	10	10	10	10

Descriptive Statistics

	Mean	Std. Deviation	N
Age	63.80	4.662	10
CD%	0.4590	0.49195	10
CNF%	8.6200	6.65078	10
RRF%	1.6900	3.04246	10

Table C: One way ANOVA comparing molecular and histological changes in different forms of myositis:

ANOVA

		Sum of Squares	df	Mean Square	F	Sig.
Age	Between Groups	873.598	3	291.199	1.937	0.138
	Within Groups	6312.859	42	150.306		
	Total	7186.457	45			
CD%	Between Groups	1.011	3	0.337	1.704	0.181
	Within Groups	8.306	42	0.198		
	Total	9.317	45			
CNF%	Between Groups	2057.369	3	685.790	2.297	0.091
	Within Groups	12538.757	42	298.542		
	Total	14596.126	45			
RRF%	Between Groups	377.810	3	125.937	1.934	0.139
	Within Groups	2734.349	42	65.104		
	Total	3112.158	45			

Robust Tests of Equality of Means

		Statistic[a]	df1	df2	Sig.
Age	Welch	6.317	3	22.460	0.003
CD%	Welch	3.326	3	18.498	0.042
CNF%	Welch	8.308	3	17.547	0.001
RRF%	Welch	0.928	3	22.667	0.443

a. Asymptotically F distributed.

Theses:

1. The degree of mtDNA deletions in muscle homogenate of myositis patients is very low (usually <1%) which is not picked up by southern blotting analysis.

2. Long-range-PCR and the specially designed specific 'common deletion PCR' are suitable methods for qualitative analysis of mtDNA deletions in myositis patients.

3. Real-time-PCR analysis documents the deletions even with very small magnitude (~ 0.01%) and hence remains the gold standard for quantatitative DNA analysis.

4. Multiple deletions and the common deletion are quite frequent in inclusion body myositis, followed by dermatomyositis and polymyositis. However, deletions could also be seen in normal cases but in very less frequency.

5. However, association of mtDNA deletions in myositis should be more important in terms of response to immuno-supressive therapy in inclusion body myositis.

6. The role of mtDNA deletions in myositis should be more important in terms of response to immuno-supressive therapy in inclusion body myositis.

7. Deletions are seen in both the COX negative and COX positive fibres in multiple-cell-real-time-PCR analysis. However, the degree of heteroplasmy of the common deletion is remarkably higher in the COX negative fibres than in the normal fibres.

8. The degree of presence of common deletion in a fibre to become COX deficient is ~ 80%.

9. There is no significant correlation between reduced biochemical COX activity and the degree of common deletion in myositis patients and normal cases.

10. Deficiency of cytochrome c oxidase in myositis is not necessarily triggered my mtDNA deletions.

11. Different forms of mitochondrial abnormalities (histological, biochemical and molecular genetic) are not significantly correlated with each other, hence, one entity does not trigger the other.

12. A sub-group with rather unusually high number of COX deficient fibres was seen and in polymyositis group, one but all patients harboured either, multiple deletions and /or the common deletion or the both.

13. No correlation was seen between the age and the degree of heteroplasmy of the common deletion even in the control group and also in myositis groups.

14. A same mechanism should promote the development of multiple mtDNA deletions in normal ageing and in all the forms of myositis. However the mechanism seems to be accentuated in IBM.

15. All the myositis patients contained COX deficient fibres and most of the patients also contained ragged-red fibres. Hence these mitochondrial defects could be considered as one of the precursors of pathogenosis in myositis.

16. Mitochondrial protein synthesis is impaired when a particular percentage of deletions in mtDNA is reached. However, the high levels of deletions in mtDNA alone do not seem to cause a severe COX deficiency and/or residual COX deficiency. This argument suggests that the defect in mitochondrial protein synthesis is predominantly by the reduction of wild-type mtDNA in affected cells.

17. The exact role of mitochondrial DNA abnormalities in pathogenosis of myositis remains still unanswered.

Acknowledgement

At the outset, I would like to thank *Prof. Dr. S. Zierz*, Director, Dept. Neurology, Martin-Luther-University Halle-Wittenberg for guiding me throughout this work. I extend my gratitude to *Prof. Dr. M. Deschauer,* Dept. Neurology, Martin-Luther-University Halle-Wittenberg for his guidance and support in conducting this work.

I would also like to extend my gratitude to everyone directly or indirectly involved with this project, especially, *Dr. P. Tacik,* Dept. Neurology, Martin-Luther-University Halle-Wittenberg for clinical characterization of patients, *Prof. Dr. H. Foth* and *Dr. F. Glahn,* Dept. Toxicology, Martin-Luther-University Halle-Wittenberg for guiding me through Real-time PCR techniques, *PD Dr. Kirches,* Dept. Neuropathology, University Magdeburg, for construction of Plasmids for Real-Time PCR and *Prof. Dr. C. Hoang-Vu* and *Mrs. K. Hammje,* ECHO laboratory, Martin-Luther-University Halle-Wittenberg for guiding me through single fibre laser micro-dissection.

This work would never have been completed without the support of my collegues fron Department of Neurology and laboratory for neuromuscular disorders. Thanks a lot *Frank, Alex, Anja, Kathleen, Thekla, Silvia, Leila, and Annette.* You are the best!

I would like to appreciate the contribution of my beloved better-half *Reshma* for her overall encouragement and guidance. Finally, a special note of thanks to my parents *Sharad* and *Dropadi,* parents-in-law *Kamal* and *Sarita*, my sister *Rubeca*, my brother-in-law *Murari,* my brothers *Lava, Padam* and *Mahendra,* my sisters-in-law *Kiran* and *Gita,* and my sweet nephews *Aryan, Abhi, Adi,* and *Rohan* for theit encouragement and support.

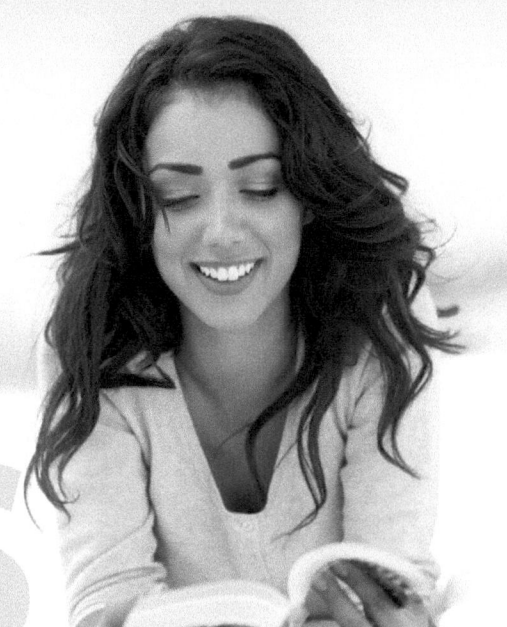

i want morebooks!

Buy your books fast and straightforward online - at one of world's fastest growing online book stores! Environmentally sound due to Print-on-Demand technologies.

Buy your books online at
www.get-morebooks.com

Kaufen Sie Ihre Bücher schnell und unkompliziert online – auf einer der am schnellsten wachsenden Buchhandelsplattformen weltweit! Dank Print-On-Demand umwelt- und ressourcenschonend produziert.

Bücher schneller online kaufen
www.morebooks.de

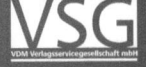 VDM Verlagsservicegesellschaft mbH
Heinrich-Böcking-Str. 6-8   Telefon: +49 681 3720 174   info@vdm-vsg.de
D - 66121 Saarbrücken   Telefax: +49 681 3720 1749   www.vdm-vsg.de

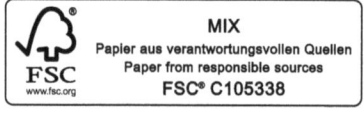

Printed by Books on Demand GmbH, Norderstedt / Germany